# Healthy Presentations

Emily P. Green

# Healthy Presentations

How to Craft Exceptional Lectures
in Medicine, the Health Professions,
and the Biomedical Sciences

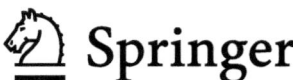 Springer

Emily P. Green
The Warren Alpert Medical School of Brown University
Providence, RI
USA

ISBN 978-3-030-72755-0        ISBN 978-3-030-72756-7    (eBook)
https://doi.org/10.1007/978-3-030-72756-7

This Springer imprint is published by the registered company Springer Nature Switzerland AG
The registered company address is: Gewerbestrasse 11, 6330 Cham, Switzerland

# Foreword

Is lecturing a thing of the past? Not if you do it right and focus on *facilitation of learning* instead of simple information transfer! As a medical educator for 30 years, and as someone who has observed countless lectures by medical faculty in my role in overseeing medical school curriculum, I am extremely excited that Dr. Emily Green's *Healthy Presentations* has come to fruition. This book fills a need for a concise, practical guide – rich with examples and options – for medical educators who are short on time but inspired to improve teaching and clarity of communication with learners.

Other available resources are typically written for the business, marketing, and corporate worlds. They do not address the specific needs of teaching in the health professions – namely complex and content-heavy presentations – and many are outdated. I have attended many of Dr. Green's faculty development workshops and lectures over the past decade and I always learn something new. Dr. Green has extensive experience in faculty development and has hands-on experience working directly with medical faculty in improving their presentations. She is an articulate and masterful communicator. Her educational background, experience in medical education, and honed skills in giving faculty feedback on their presentations make her uniquely suited to addressing the need for an up-to-date, concise, well-written guide for medical educators.

Dr. Green shares her skills in faculty development with the medical and health professions community in *Healthy Presentations*. Whether you are just beginning to craft new lectures, or you have been doing this for a long time, I am certain you will find invaluable advice and concrete examples in this book that you will be able to readily put into action.

While the national trend in medical education is directed away from traditional lecturing, I would argue, as Dr. Green does in this book, that well-designed, increasingly interactive, and clearly communicated presentations are here to stay. The changes in medical education that have been accelerated by the COVID-19 pandemic starkly outline the challenges of distant, depersonalized learning. In a very timely chapter, Dr. Green addresses ways to actively engage learners in virtual and asynchronous teaching modules.

In another timely chapter, Dr. Green outlines approaches that medical educators can use to assure that their presentations are inclusive and anti-racist. Dr. Green has been working closely with our medical faculty in putting these approaches into practice. She shares this expertise in a straightforward practical fashion using concrete examples. This unique perspective will be much appreciated by medical educators seeking to develop inclusive teaching and learning materials.

I learned much of what I know over the years by teaching and observing faculty members, fine-tuning the art of interactive teaching. I wish a guide like this had been available to me when I was starting out. I learned the hard way – by trial and error – the latter of which is far less beneficial to our learners. Dr. Green has accumulated a wealth of knowledge that she shares in *Healthy Presentations* that will be extremely helpful to medical educators. Enjoy!

Luba Dumenco, MD, MEHP, FACP
Associate Professor of Medical Science
The Warren Alpert Medical School of Brown University
Providence, RI, USA

# Acknowledgments

I owe an enormous debt of gratitude to the medical faculty of The Warren Alpert Medical School of Brown University with whom I have worked over the last 15 years. Thank you for granting me the privilege of watching your presentations, and for being brave and vulnerable enough to allow me to critique them.

A special thank you to Dr. Luba Dumenco for granting me extraordinary access to her lecture content. She is an outstanding educator and a highly talented presenter who has won many teaching awards over the years. This book would not be possible without her.

Thank you to Drs. Kristina Monteiro, Robert Tubbs, Allan Tunkel, and Jordan White for access to their lecture and scholarly content.

Thank you to Dr. Jason Hack for the "presenter as Instagram star" metaphor used in Chap. 3.

Thank you to Dr. Wael Asaad for the mushroom metaphor used in Chap. 5, Example 5.24.

Thank you to Dr. Angela Anderson for the "slide sorter" tip mentioned in Chap. 5.

A big thank you to Philip G. Rickards, the original presenter!

Finally, all my love to Bob, Charlotte, Alice, and Leo Green, my extraordinarily supportive husband and three wonderful children.

# Contents

**1   Quality Matters**................................................   1
   1.1   The Current State of Affairs................................   1
   1.2   My Confession........................................   2
   1.3   Quality Matters ......................................   3
   References............................................   6

**2   Myth-Busting**..................................................   7
   References............................................  11

**3   Crafting a Talk** ...............................................  13
   3.1   Understanding Your Learners............................  13
   3.2   Defining Your Core Concepts ...........................  14
   3.3   Use of Active Verbs ..................................  15
   3.4   Identifying Appropriate Teaching Strategies .................  15
   3.5   Beware the Inherited Slides ............................  16
   3.6   Beginnings .........................................  17
   3.7   Middles ...........................................  20
   3.8   Endings ...........................................  25
   References............................................  26

**4   Incorporating Opportunities for Active Learning** ...............  27
   4.1   Defining Active Learning...............................  27
   4.2   Use of Questions ....................................  28
   4.3   Workshop Elements ..................................  30
   4.4   Mini-Assignments ...................................  32
   4.5   Case-Based Learning..................................  33
   References............................................  35

**5   The Basics of Slide Design** .....................................  37
   5.1   Anatomy of a Presentation.............................  37
   5.2   Common Slide Design.................................  39
   5.3   Assertion-Evidence Design .............................  40
   References............................................  61

**6   Reviewing Slides for Diversity and Inclusion** . . . . . . . . . . . . . . . . .   63
  6.1   Diversity of Images . . . . . . . . . . . . . . . . . . . . . . . . . . . . . . . . .   64
  6.2   Inclusivity of Language and Terminology . . . . . . . . . . . . . . . . . .   67
  6.3   Review of Citations . . . . . . . . . . . . . . . . . . . . . . . . . . . . . . . . .   68
  6.4   Race as a Risk Factor . . . . . . . . . . . . . . . . . . . . . . . . . . . . . . . .   69
  6.5   Prevalence by Racial Category  . . . . . . . . . . . . . . . . . . . . . . . . .   73
  6.6   Range of Possible Edits . . . . . . . . . . . . . . . . . . . . . . . . . . . . . .   75
  References . . . . . . . . . . . . . . . . . . . . . . . . . . . . . . . . . . . . . . . . . . .   79

**7   The Delivery** . . . . . . . . . . . . . . . . . . . . . . . . . . . . . . . . . . . . . . . .   81
  7.1   In Preparation (Before)  . . . . . . . . . . . . . . . . . . . . . . . . . . . . . .   81
  7.2   In the Moment (During) . . . . . . . . . . . . . . . . . . . . . . . . . . . . . .   83
  7.3   Post-Delivery (After) . . . . . . . . . . . . . . . . . . . . . . . . . . . . . . . .   84
  References . . . . . . . . . . . . . . . . . . . . . . . . . . . . . . . . . . . . . . . . . . .   85

**8   Presenting Virtually** . . . . . . . . . . . . . . . . . . . . . . . . . . . . . . . . . .   87
  8.1   General Tips . . . . . . . . . . . . . . . . . . . . . . . . . . . . . . . . . . . . . .   88
  8.2   Considerations for In-Person, Recorded Lectures . . . . . . . . . . . .   90
  8.3   Considerations for Remote Presenting to an In-Person Group . . . .   92
  8.4   Considerations for Fully Remote Presenting . . . . . . . . . . . . . . . .   95
  References . . . . . . . . . . . . . . . . . . . . . . . . . . . . . . . . . . . . . . . . . . .  100

**9   Implementing Change** . . . . . . . . . . . . . . . . . . . . . . . . . . . . . . . .  101

**Index** . . . . . . . . . . . . . . . . . . . . . . . . . . . . . . . . . . . . . . . . . . . . . . . .  105

# References

Acquaviva KD, Mintz M. Perspective: are we teaching racial profiling? The dangers of subjective determinations of race and ethnicity in case presentations. Acad Med. 2010;85(4):702–5.

Alley M. The craft of scientific presentations: critical steps to succeed and critical errors to avoid. 2nd ed; 2013.

Anderson LW, Bloom BS. A taxonomy for learning, teaching, and assessing: a revision of Bloom's taxonomy of educational objectives. Longman; 2001.

Anderson MR, Moscou S, Fulchon C, Neuspiel DR. The role of race in the clinical presentation. Family Medicine-Kansas City. 2001;33(6):430–4.

Atkinson C. Beyond bullet points: using Microsoft PowerPoint to create presentations that inform, motivate, and inspire (Bpg-other). Microsoft Press; 2005.

Barr RB, Tagg J. From teaching to learning—a new paradigm for undergraduate education. Change: The Magazine of Higher Learning. 1995;27(6):12–26.

Bennett C. Racial categories used in the decennial censuses, 1790 to the present. Gov Inf Q. 2000;17(2):161–80.

Bloom BS. Taxonomy of educational objectives: the classification of educational goals. Handbook 1: cognitive domain. New York: David McKay Co. Inc.; 1956.

Braun LT, Zwaan L, Kiesewetter J, Fischer MR, Schmidmaier R. Diagnostic errors by medical students: results of a prospective qualitative study. BMC Med Educ. 2017;17(1):191.

Brondolo E, Love EE, Pencille M, Schoenthaler A, Ogedegbe G. Racism and hypertension: a review of the empirical evidence and implications for clinical practice. Am J Hypertens. 2011;24(5):518–29.

Brown A. The changing categories the US has used to measure race. Pew Research Center. 2015;7(3):15.

Brown PC, Roediger HL III, McDaniel MA. Make it stick. Harvard University Press; 2014.

Bruner J. Life as narrative. Soc Res: An international quarterly. 2004;71(3):691–710.

Carvalho JAMD, Wood CH, Andrade FCD. Estimating the stability of census-based racial/ethnic classifications: the case of Brazil. Popul Stud. 2004;58(3):331–43.

Dror I, Schmidt P, O'connor L. A cognitive perspective on technology enhanced learning in medical training: great opportunities, pitfalls and challenges. Med Teach. 2011;33(4):291–6.

Dror IE, Stevenage SV, Ashworth AR. Helping the cognitive system learn: exaggerating distinctiveness and uniqueness. Appl Cogn Psychol. 2008;22(4):573–84.

Duarte N. Slide: ology: the art and science of creating great presentations, vol. 1. Sebastapol: O'Reilly Media; 2008.

Dunlosky J, Rawson KA, Marsh EJ, Nathan MJ, Willingham DT. Improving students' learning with effective learning techniques: promising directions from cognitive and educational psychology. Psychol Sci Public Interest. 2013;14(1):4–58.

Easton G. How medical teachers use narratives in lectures: a qualitative study. BMC Med Educ. 2016;16(1):3.

Fornari A, Poznanski A, editors. How-to guide for active learning. International Association of Medical Science Educators.

Garner JK, Alley MP, Sawarynski LE, Wolfe KL, Zappe SE. Assertion-evidence slides appear to lead to better comprehension and recall of more complex concepts. In: ASEE annual conference and exposition, conference proceedings; 2011.

Garner J, Alley M. How the design of presentation slides affects audience comprehension: a case for the assertion-evidence approach. Int J Eng Educ. 2013;29(6):1564–79.

Goddu AP, O'Conor KJ, Lanzkron S, Saheed MO, Saha S, Peek ME, et al. Do words matter? Stigmatizing language and the transmission of bias in the medical record. J Gen Intern Med. 2018;33(5):685–91.

Graber ML, Franklin N, Gordon R. Diagnostic error in internal medicine. Arch Intern Med. 2005;165(13):1493–9.

Guidelines for promoting a bias-free curriculum [Internet]. Vagelos College of Physicians and Surgeons. Vagelos College of Physicians and Surgeons; 2018 [cited 2019Oct28]. Available from: https://www.ps.columbia.edu/education/student-resources/honor-code-and-policies/guidelines-promoting-bias-free-curriculum

Hern A. Trolls exploit zoom privacy settings as app gains popularity, GUARDIAN (Mar. 27, 2020 8:23 AM), https://www.theguardian.com/technology/2020/mar/27/trolls-zoom-privacy-settings-covid-19-lockdown, FORBES (Mar. 27, 2020 11:19 AM).

Hoffman KM, Trawalter S, Axt JR, Oliver MN. Racial bias in pain assessment and treatment recommendations, and false beliefs about biological differences between blacks and whites. Proc Natl Acad Sci. 2016;113(16):4296–301.

Ikonne U, Campbell AM, Whelihan KE, Bay RC, Lewis JH. Exodus from the classroom: student perceptions, lecture capture technology, and the inception of on-demand preclinical medical education. J Am Osteopath Assoc. 2018;118(12):813–23.

Jackson-Richards D, Pandya AG, editors. Dermatology atlas for skin of color. Berlin, Heidelberg: Springer; 2014.

Kernbach S, Bresciani S. 10 years after Tufte's "cognitive style of PowerPoint": synthesizing its constraining qualities. In: 2013 17th international conference on information visualisation. IEEE; 2013, July. p. 345–50.

King-O'Riain RC. Counting on the Celtic Tiger' adding ethnic census categories in the Republic of Ireland. Ethnicities. 2007;7(4):516–42.

Knowles MS. Self-directed learning: a guide for learners and teachers. Chicago: Association Press; 1975.

Krishnan A, Rabinowitz M, Ziminsky A, Scott SM, Chretien KC. Addressing race, culture, and structural inequality in medical education: a guide for revising teaching cases. Acad Med. 2019;94(4):550–5.

Krupat E, Wormwood J, Schwartzstein RM, Richards JB. Avoiding premature closure and reaching diagnostic accuracy: some key predictive factors. Med Educ. 2017;51(11):1127–37.

Lang JM. Small teaching: everyday lessons from the science of learning. San Francisco: Wiley; 2016.

Marte D. Can a woman of color trust medical education? Acad Med. 2019;94(7):928–30.

Matson CC, Beck LA, Rajasekaran SK. Using language that reflects who is the center of our care. Acad Med. 2019;94(9):1400.

Mayer RE. Multimedia learning. Cambridge: Cambridge University Press; 2009.

McKevitt C, Morgan M. Illness doesn't belong to us. J R Soc Med. 1997;90(9):491–5.

Merriam SB, Caffarella R, Baumgartner S. Learning in adulthood: a comprehensive guide. 3rd ed. San Francisco: Jossey-Bass; 2007.

Michael J. Where's the evidence that active learning works? Adv Physiol Educ. 2006.

Mohanty M, Yaqub W. Towards seamless authentication for zoom-based online teaching and meeting. arXiv preprint arXiv:200510553. 2020.

Morrison M. How to create a better research poster in less time. 2019. https://www.youtube.com/watch?v=1RwJbhkCA58. Accessed 9.23.20.

Nathans-Kelly T, Nicometo CG. Slide rules: design, build, and archive presentations in the engineering and technical fields, vol. 3. Wiley; 2014.

Prince M. Does active learning work? A review of the research. J Eng Educ. 2004;93(3):223–31.

Prober CG, Heath C. Lecture halls without lectures—a proposal for medical education. N Engl J Med. 2012;366(18):1657–9.

Reynolds G. Presentation Zen design: a simple visual approach to presenting in today's world. Pearson Education; 2014.

Rideout M, Held M, Holmes AV. The didactic makeover: keep it short, active, relevant. Pediatrics. 2016;138(1).

Rossiter M. Understanding adult development as narrative. New Dir Adult Contin Educ. 1999;1999(84):77–85.

Sandefur GD, Campbell ME, Eggerling-Boeck J. Racial and ethnic identification, official classifications, and health disparities. Critical perspectives on racial and ethnic differences in health in late life. 2004:25–52.

Schraeder TL. Physician communication: connecting with patients, peers, and the public. Oxford University Press; 2019.

Taylor SSC, Serrano AMA, Kelly AP, Lim H. Taylor and Kelly's dermatology for skin of color. McGraw-Hill; 2016.

Thomas PA, Kern DE, Hughes MT, Chen BY, editors. Curriculum development for medical education: a six-step approach. JHU Press; 2016.

Trent M, Dooley DG, Dougé J. The impact of racism on child and adolescent health. Pediatrics. 2019;144(2):e20191765.

Tsai J, Ucik L, Baldwin N, Hasslinger C, George P. Race matters? Examining and rethinking race portrayal in preclinical medical education. Acad Med. 2016;91(7):916–20.

Tsai J, Crawford-Roberts A. A call for critical race theory in medical education. Acad Med. 2017;92(8):1072–3.

Tufte ER. The cognitive style of PowerPoint. New York: AP/Wide World Photos; 2003.

Yudell M, Roberts D, DeSalle R, Tishkoff S. Taking race out of human genetics. Science. 2016;351(6273):564–5.

Vyas DA, Eisenstein LG, Jones DS. Hidden in plain sight—reconsidering the use of race correction in clinical algorithms. N Engl J Med. 2020;383:874.

Wang J, Antonenko PD. Instructor presence in instructional video: effects on visual attention, recall, and perceived learning. Comput Hum Behav. 2017;71:79–89.

Wang J, Antonenko P, Dawson K. Does visual attention to the instructor in online video affect learning and learner perceptions? An eye-tracking analysis. Comput Educ. 2020;146:103779.

Wiggins GP, McTighe J. Understanding by Design. Alexandria: Association for Supervision and Curriculum Development; 1998.

Williams DR, Lawrence JA, Davis BA. Racism and health: evidence and needed research. Annu Rev Public Health. 2019;40:105–25.

Wolff M, Wagner MJ, Poznanski S, Schiller J, Santen S. Not another boring lecture: engaging learners with active learning techniques. J Emerg Med. 2015;48(1):85–93.

Woolf K, Cave J, McManus IC, Dacre JE. It gives you an understanding you can't get from any book'. The relationship between medical students' and doctors' personal illness experiences and their performance: a qualitative and quantitative study. BMC Med Educ. 2007;7(1):50.

# Chapter 1
# Quality Matters

**Abstract**
This introductory chapter makes the case that traditional academic presentations in medicine and the health professions do not adequately focus on the facilitation of learning, and that improved lecture quality could have an enormous impact on both individual learners and the professions themselves. *Healthy presentations* are defined as ones that assist our learners in effectively and efficiently comprehending and retaining information. Overviews of subsequent chapters are provided.

## 1.1 The Current State of Affairs

We all know by now that there is a problem with the format of traditional academic lectures [1–5]. Each of us – clinician, biomedical researcher, medical educator– has sat through hundreds, if not thousands of hours of lecture. And each of those hours probably included tens, if not hundreds, of slides.

Collectively we are thoroughly exhausted by the endless parade of headings and bullet points, tired of sitting through another tedious brain-dump given by a student, resident, or colleague. These lectures seem far more about what the lecturer wants to say, than they are about what we in the audience need and want to learn. We divide our attention between the glow of the big screen and the smaller glow of our phones, our thumbs swiping and clicking as the presentation drones on in the background.

We tune in occasionally for a pearl of wisdom or two, but we will look the topic up later if the need really arises. If the topic is of particular interest, or if there will be some kind of assessment at the conclusion of the talk, we try to follow along, attempting to glean major concepts from the progression of slides.

E. P. Green, *Healthy Presentations*, https://doi.org/10.1007/978-3-030-72756-7_1

Even more occasionally, a charismatic speaker will capture our attention and the energy in the room will shift. The talk is well-crafted, relevant to the audience at hand, and perfectly paced. The speaker is articulate and engaging, master of his or her content. We leave feeling inspired, informed, and even refreshed. Such is the power of a good lecture. Powerful, yet so rare.

## 1.2   My Confession

As an educator, I probably should not say this, but *I love a good lecture*. In medicine and health professions education, we rely on them too much as a relatively low-resource option to educate large groups of learners. We fail to consider alternate modes of instruction that may be more appropriate for particular content. We also do not provide those individuals doing the presenting with any formal training in how to do it well. But a good lecture, on an appropriately targeted topic, is a thing of beauty.

Lectures are the perfect modality for overviews and introductions, for providing background information and foundational frameworks for subsequent content, for convincing an audience of a particular point of view. Succinct lectures can report results, highlight advances, and establish best practices. Engaging lectures can launch discussions, inform skill-acquisition, and stimulate collaboration. Inclusive lectures can combat bias, correct misinformation, and create community. *Exceptional* lectures effectively and efficiently facilitate learning.

I am an educator by training, and I have made my career in medical education. As part of my work, I have watched thousands of lectures and presentations. My absolute favorite part of my job is the talk-review service I run for faculty members. Faculty come to me with presentations they are doing for the first time, and presentations they do repeatedly for different groups of learners. They come with lectures for Year 1 medical students, and presentations for national conferences. Their presentations are 10 minutes, 60 minutes, or even 90 minutes long. Some faculty have an intense fear of public speaking. Others are seasoned presenters who just want a new set of eyes to take a look at their slides. I get to watch presentations on medical abortion, genetics counseling, vaping, treatments for opioid addiction, disability advocacy, care of transgender patients, development of a mock code program, suicide prevention, colorectal surgical procedures...the list is endless.

I have learned so much over the years, and feel so honored to help faculty make concrete improvements to their teaching and presenting. I am passionate about these improvements because *I firmly believe that we can draw a direct connection from good presentations to the learning they facilitate*. If we improve our lectures, we improve the ability of our learners to understand and retain the information contained within them. From learner comprehension and retention, we can draw indirect, but indelible, lines to the quality of patient care, to the reduction of medical error, and to the wellness of our physician workforce.

## 1.3 Quality Matters

Educational psychologists agree that knowledge is constructed [6–11]. Our learners come to us, not as blank slates, but with an array of experience and understanding that provides a starting point for further learning. Lectures that facilitate learning guide learners as they organize new information, construct mental models of that information, and then integrate it with their prior knowledge. Even if our learners are our peers (or indeed our supervisors, mentors, or professional idols), we have a responsibility to help them tap into their experience and knowledge, and to build upon it.

The goal of every presentation is to help our learners construct new knowledge [12]. As presenters, we facilitate an active meaning-making process that is essential for deep understanding. *The facilitation of learning is perhaps more essential in medicine and the health professions than in any other discipline.*

In his essay, "The Cognitive Style of PowerPoint: Pitching Out Corrupts Within," Edward Tufte (2006) makes a powerful argument against the use of PowerPoint as a communication tool within the sciences. Though he refers specifically to engineering, much of his argument applies to the biomedical sciences, and to presentation software programs other than PowerPoint, as well. According to Tufte, the default settings of PowerPoint (headings with lists of bulleted items and sub-items) do not allow learners to assess the presenter's reasoning, the scope of the data presented, or the relationships between data points, other than basic membership and hierarchy. "Information stacked in time makes it difficult to understand context and evaluate relationships" (p. 5).

Tufte goes on to dissect a particular set of slides used by NASA in 2003 when the space shuttle Columbia was damaged upon its launch, and engineers back on the ground attempted to assess the danger posed by re-entry into the Earth's atmosphere [5]. As we know, the Columbia ultimately exploded, killing all seven astronauts on board. Tufte, and indeed the Columbia Accident Investigation Board, implicates PowerPoint-based communication as a contributing factor in these deaths.

It is a stretch to say that one poorly designed lecture, on recognizing stroke for example, could be directly linked to a particular patient's death. Medical education is not that simple or linear in nature. There are of course many sources of a physician's knowledge about stroke, many of which are experiential and do not have their roots in lecture-based teaching at all.

However, given the packed schedules of medical students, nurses, physician assistants, residents, and attendings, and given the sheer number of hours of lecture that each watches throughout their professional training, is it so farfetched to say that improved presentations could improve learning? That improved learning could prevent academic struggle and hours spent on redundant study? That reducing academic struggle and unnecessary content-review could free up time to catch up on sleep, learn new things, deepen understanding, and build expertise?

Let us consider for a moment a hypothetical second-year medical student, "Ginny," who sits through an average of three hours of lecture each day. She views some lectures as recordings from her apartment, but she has trouble paying attention on her own, so she likes to attend in person most of the time. Ginny has come to realize that prior to each exam she needs to review each lecture a second, and ideally a third time, before she feels that she thoroughly understands and remembers the material.

United States Medical Licensing Exam (USMLE) Step 1, the first of her high-stakes comprehensive licensing exams, is quickly approaching and Ginny knows that she has big knowledge gaps from some of the basic science courses in Year 1. Last year she found BioChem and Microbiology particularly difficult. Ginny now agrees with the saying about medical education being like "drinking from a firehose" with so much content coming at her all at the same time. The medical school's learning specialist told Ginny that she is getting lost in all of the details, and that she needs to be better able to "see the forest through the trees."

Ginny is very worried about being able to adequately prepare for USMLE Step 1 within the six weeks provided by the medical school. Based on several of her Year 1 exam scores, it appears that she did not learn the material very well the first time around, so she worries that Step-prep is going to feel like starting from scratch. Ginny really needs to spend more time practicing for the upcoming objective structured clinical exam (OSCE), but she just does not think she can spare the hours.

Now consider for a moment the harried resident that Ginny will eventually become. She has experienced many additional lectures since her days as a medical student – most of them as poorly designed as the ones she sat through in medical school. She takes fewer exams now, but still has trouble digesting information presented in lecture form. She still has to spend time looking up information in other ways, from other sources, and she feels like she has not slept in days. Ginny's relationships are suffering because these days all she seems to do is work and study.

How different might Ginny's situation be if those many lectures she attended over the years had been…better? If Ginny had found it easier to learn from them the first time they were delivered? If the lectures had helped her construct new knowledge in such a way that she did not need to review each of them multiple times in order to "see" those foundational concepts through the myriad of details provided? If presenters had attended to her need to learn large amounts of content efficiently, and with effective cognitive investment? [10, 13, 14]. If Step-prep had consisted of review, not primary learning? Might Ginny now be better rested, less isolated, and more adept at forming diagnoses?

If her education had included better lectures, could Ginny now be, in essence, a better doctor?

*Taken in totality, the impact of improved presenting on learning is potentially immense* [1, 3, 10]. Learning things better, in more depth, and more efficiently, could play an important, if indirect, role in improving patient care, preventing medical error, and reducing physician burnout.

Presentation quality matters. As clinicians, educators, and researchers, it is our responsibility to guide our learners as they construct new knowledge within very limited timeframes, and highly pressurized environments. *Healthy presentations* are ones that help our learners to effectively and efficiently comprehend and retain the information we deliver.

Once you have decided that a lecture or presentation is the appropriate teaching modality for your particular content, what are the important considerations to take into account? How can we engage our learners, lead them through the major concepts we have identified as essential, and facilitate the learning process?

**How can we create *Healthy Presentations?***
In Chap. 2, I review four common myths about lectures that have prevented us from translating our collective presentation-fatigue into presentation-reform.

In Chap. 3, I discuss presentation construction, how to engage learners right off the bat, and keep them engaged throughout a talk.

In Chap. 4, I expand on the idea of learner engagement and review techniques to integrate active learning opportunities into a presentation.

In Chap. 5, I present the complete anatomy of a presentation, which includes more than just your verbal delivery. I also review sets of rules and opportunities for improved slide design.

In Chap. 6, I discuss the importance of reviewing your slides for inclusivity and bias as part of antiracist teaching practices. I provide practical tips and examples of changes you can make.

In Chap. 7, I discuss lecture delivery, and what to do before, during, and after you present.

In Chap. 8, I provide a number of tips for engaging learners during *virtual* presentations.

In Chap. 9, I end this book with advice about implementing change. I review how to engage in the process of revising existing presentations, and of developing new and different presentations going forward.

This book is a call to action. I recognize that your time is limited, and that you may have had little or no formal training on how to lecture or teach. However, lectures are not going anywhere, especially in medicine and health professions education. Lecture quality can have real down-stream consequences for our learners and future colleagues, so it is our responsibility to focus on making changes to our presentations that will improve the learner experience. This book is designed to help us do just that.

The information I include here is based on my training as an educator, and my years of experience working with both medical students and medical faculty. The tips and suggestions I provide are intentionally specific and concrete. While broadly based in current understanding of cognitive psychology and the science of teaching and learning, *this book is meant to be, above all else, a practical resource for busy clinicians who seek to improve their instructional practice.*

### Summary Points

- Lectures are an important educational tool, but we need to improve their quality.
- Traditional academic presentations in medicine and the health professions do not adequately focus on the facilitation of learning.
- Higher quality presentations could have an enormous impact on individual learners and on the health professions themselves.

## References

1. Alley M. The craft of scientific presentations: critical steps to succeed and critical errors to avoid. 2nd ed. New York: Springer; 2013.
2. Kernbach S, Bresciani S. 10 years after Tufte's "cognitive style of PowerPoint": synthesizing its constraining qualities. In: 2013 17th international conference on information visualisation. IEEE; 2013, July. p. 345–50.
3. Nathans-Kelly T, Nicometo CG. Slide rules: design, build, and archive presentations in the engineering and technical fields, vol. 3. Hoboken: Wiley; 2014.
4. Reynolds G. Presentation Zen design: a simple visual approach to presenting in today's world. Berkeley: Pearson Education; 2014.
5. Tufte ER. The cognitive style of PowerPoint. New York: AP/Wide World Photos; 2003.
6. Barr RB, Tagg J. From teaching to learning—a new paradigm for undergraduate education. Change: The Magazine of Higher Learning. 1995;27(6):12–26.
7. Brown PC, Roediger HL III, McDaniel MA. Make it stick. Harvard University Press; 2014.
8. Dunlosky J, Rawson KA, Marsh EJ, Nathan MJ, Willingham DT. Improving students' learning with effective learning techniques: promising directions from cognitive and educational psychology. Psychol Sci Public Interest. 2013;14(1):4–58.
9. Lang JM. Small teaching: everyday lessons from the science of learning. San Francisco: Wiley; 2016.
10. Mayer RE. Multimedia learning. Cambridge: Cambridge University Press; 2009.
11. Merriam SB, Caffarella R, Baumgartner S. Learning in adulthood: a comprehensive guide. 3rd ed. San Francisco: Jossey-Bass; 2007.
12. Wiggins GP, McTighe J. Understanding by design. Alexandria: Association for Supervision and Curriculum Development; 1998.
13. Dror I, Schmidt P, O'connor L. A cognitive perspective on technology enhanced learning in medical training: great opportunities, pitfalls and challenges. Med Teach. 2011;33(4):291–6.
14. Dror IE, Stevenage SV, Ashworth AR. Helping the cognitive system learn: exaggerating distinctiveness and uniqueness. Appl Cogn Psychol. 2008;22(4):573–84.

# Chapter 2
# Myth-Busting

**Abstract**
This chapter identifies and counters four common myths about biomedical presentations. Barriers to change include mythology around the definition of "professional" presentations, perceived limitations of content-dense presentations, audiences' unacknowledged need for structure and guidance, and a focus on teaching rather than learning. Facilitation of learning is the central goal of all *healthy presentations*.

If traditional academic lectures are so bad, and good presentations are so rare, why is there not more of a movement for change in medical and health professions education? In this chapter, I will address four pervasive myths that I believe act as barriers to positive change.

---

MYTH #1: *Traditional presentations may be boring, but they are professional.*

---

There are accepted norms for presentations within different professions, and within different areas of academia. In the biomedical sciences and health professions education, these norms tend to include dense, text-based slide decks, presented in a traditional, unidirectional (faculty-to-learner) manner. While professionally acceptable, we should aim higher. As currently designed, our presentations may be falling short of their ultimate goal – to facilitate learning for our audiences.

For many people, the idea of public speaking, even to small or familiar audiences, can cause a great deal of anxiety. And when we are anxious, we tend to avoid risk and stick with what is familiar. While it is true that it can feel very risky to present your content in ways that differ from the norm, we need to widen our definition of "professional." Professional and serious does not need to be boring [1, 2]. There are many ways to present dense content in such a way that your audience takes you, and your work, seriously. Defaulting to traditional slide design, and to a pedantic, predictable delivery, does not make you more or less professional. But it does act as an impediment to efficient knowledge construction on the part of your learners. *Presentations should be seen as "professional" when they successfully further the cognitive development of learners.*

We are all tired of being on the receiving end of traditional presentations. Now we need to channel that presentation-fatigue into changes to our *own* presentations, when *we* are the ones who are in front of an audience.

> MYTH #2: *Biomedical presentations are so rich with content that the only way to get all of the information across is via traditional text-based slides.*

While biomedical presentations are necessarily dense, it is *not* necessary for them to be designed exclusively in the traditional fashion, using presentation software default settings [1–5]. These default settings perpetuate the use of brief, centered headings followed by bulleted lists of undifferentiated text. Just because scientific content does not lend itself to slides of beautiful sunsets, or artfully arranged rock piles on a sandy beach (Example 2.1), that does not mean we can ignore important aspects of good slide design.

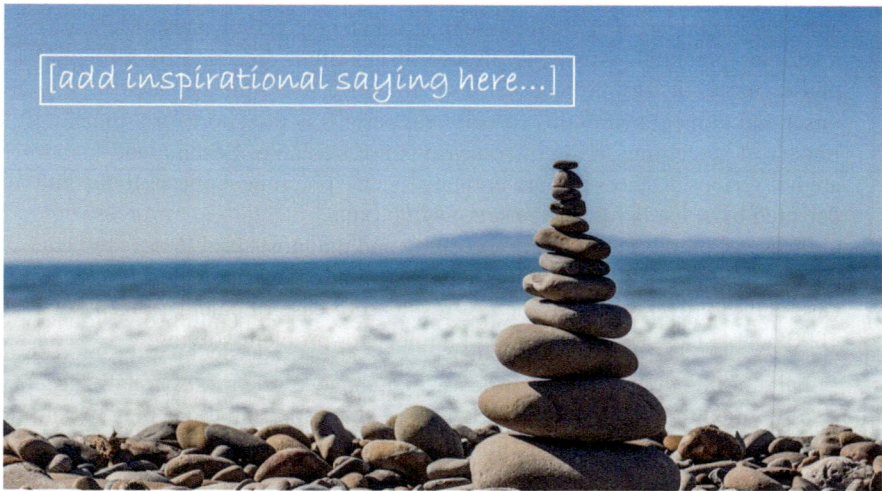

**Example 2.1**  Use of beautiful imagery, inappropriate for biomedical presentations

*We do not need to choose between well-designed slides and content-rich slides. While biomedical presentations may not include slides that consist of inspirational sayings and images of zen piles on a sandy beach, we can create slides that go beyond traditional text-only bulleted lists, and that are beautiful in their educational utility.*

Myth #2 is particularly damaging because the importance of slide design goes beyond visual appeal [4, 6]. Good slide design can help to facilitate learning by eliminating distractions, easing learners' "cognitive load," [7–9] and on a very basic level, keeping learners engaged.

Throughout this book I will talk often about learner "engagement" as foundational to facilitating learning. It is common sense that learners must be engaged and paying attention in order to learn. Slide design that is appealing, that engages the eye and the mind, is an important first step, but we cannot stop there. We need to lead our learners through our material, and augment our presentations with teaching strategies that facilitate "active" learning (see Chap. 4).

We do not need photos of rocks on a beach to make scientific presentations more visually appealing, but we do need to make changes to what and how we present in order to more efficiently and effectively facilitate learning.

---

MYTH #3: *My audience members are highly intelligent and may even be experts in their own right. I do not have to worry about them being able to follow my presentation.*

---

We never want to pander to our audience. And we certainly do not want to "dumb down" our content. However, everyone wants a talk that is organized, targeted appropriately, and easy to understand. Everyone wants a talk that flows seamlessly from topic to topic. Everyone wants, and benefits from, a talk they can follow [1, 3, 9]. So it is up to us to lead and guide. It is up to us to hold those metaphorical hands throughout each of our presentations in order to help our learners make meaningful connections, and to transform content into knowledge.

---

MYTH #4 (the Biggest Myth of All): *Teaching is about the teacher.*

---

Spoiler alert – it is not. The only measure of good teaching is the learning it facilitates. As a teacher, it is not enough to "cover" content [10]. It is not enough to take all of that wonderful information and knowledge you have in your brain, put it on some slides, and think for one minute that you are finished, that you have done your job as an educator. You have not. Teaching is not about the teacher, it is about the learning that teacher facilitates in the minds of others [11].

**Key Point**
Good teaching is less about the performance of the teacher, and more about the learning it facilitates.

Barr and Tagg (1995) discuss a movement from the traditional "instruction paradigm," in which institutions of higher education are arranged with teachers and teaching at their center, to a new "learning paradigm" that "ends the lecture's privileged position, honoring in its place whatever approaches serve best to prompt learning of particular knowledge by particular students" (p. 14). Medical and health professions education will always rightly prioritize patient care. However, institutions of medical and health professions education are overdue for a movement of their own – one that redefines teaching by the learning that it facilitates [10]. "Though considerations about what to teach and how to teach it may dominate our thinking as a matter of habit, the challenge is to focus first on the desired learnings from which appropriate teaching will logically follow" (Wiggins, p. 14).

The fact that teaching is not about the teacher, and lecturing is not about the lecturer, also means that your slides are not for you, they are for your audience. We often find ourselves designing slides to use as cue cards or as a teleprompter [6]. We include text as a reminder of what to say and how to say it. Those vague headings signal content transitions – they are as much for us as for our learners. Without all of this text, we worry that we will become anxious, lose our place, or forget to mention something important. Unfortunately, these fears lead us to create traditional text-heavy slides with little variation and even less potential for learner engagement.

Slides-as-cue-cards is a misuse of an educational tool. Your slides are not prompts for your verbal delivery. They are not the public representation of your knowledge, your work, or your professional accomplishments. Your slides are for your learners. They are a tool to facilitate learning. As such, they should be developed with the learner, not the teacher, in mind.

Lectures have traditionally been seen as teacher-centered endeavors in that you are the one doing the majority of the talking. However, there are ways to design presentations such that learners, and their personal knowledge creation, are at the center. Our goal is to move from teacher-centered presentations, to presentations that are learner-centered and teacher-delivered.

While the myths discussed here are pervasive, they should not prevent us from making changes to the way we present. We need to challenge assumptions about how and why we present the way we do in medicine and the health professions. The facilitation of learning is the single, and central goal of a *healthy presentation*. If we keep learning as our guiding principle, we will be well on our way to creating better, more engaging, and more effective, presentations.

**Summary Points**
- Common myths about biomedical presentations act as barriers to change.
- Presentations should be seen as "professional" when they successfully further the cognitive development of learners.
- Presentations with dense biomedical content do not have to rely solely on traditional teaching strategies and text-based materials.

- All presentations should be organized and delivered such that the audience finds it easy to follow along.
- As educators, we should transition from a focus on teachers and teaching, to a focus on learners and learning.

# References

1. Alley M. The craft of scientific presentations: critical steps to succeed and critical errors to avoid. 2nd ed. New York: Springer; 2013.
2. Nathans-Kelly T, Nicometo CG. Slide rules: design, build, and archive presentations in the engineering and technical fields, vol. 3. Hoboken: Wiley; 2014.
3. Atkinson C. Beyond bullet points: using Microsoft PowerPoint to create presentations that inform, motivate, and inspire (Bpg-other). Microsoft Press; 2005.
4. Reynolds G. Presentation Zen design: a simple visual approach to presenting in today's world. Berkeley: Pearson Education; 2014.
5. Tufte ER. The cognitive style of PowerPoint. New York: AP/Wide World Photos; 2003.
6. Duarte N. Slide: ology: the art and science of creating great presentations, vol. 1. Sebastapol: O'Reilly Media; 2008.
7. Dror I, Schmidt P, O'connor L. A cognitive perspective on technology enhanced learning in medical training: great opportunities, pitfalls and challenges. Med Teach. 2011;33(4):291–6.
8. Dror IE, Stevenage SV, Ashworth AR. Helping the cognitive system learn: exaggerating distinctiveness and uniqueness. Appl Cogn Psychol. 2008;22(4):573–84.
9. Mayer RE. Multimedia learning. Cambridge: Cambridge University Press; 2009.
10. Wiggins GP, McTighe J. Understanding by Design. Alexandria: Association for Supervision and Curriculum Development; 1998.
11. Barr RB, Tagg J. From teaching to learning—a new paradigm for undergraduate education. Change: The Magazine of Higher Learning. 1995;27(6):12–26.

# Chapter 3
# Crafting a Talk

**Abstract**
This chapter reviews a series of steps to take prior to slide creation, including asking questions about your learners, identifying core concepts, and selecting appropriate teaching strategies. It details the dangers of using inherited slides, and considerations for crafting effective beginnings, middles, and ends of presentations. *Healthy presentations* are defined as appropriately targeted to the audience, designed to advance specific learning objectives, and conveyed in a way that facilitates comprehension and retention. Readers are encouraged to practice "instructional empathy" as part of learner-centered presentation development.

When crafting a talk, there are a number of steps to take *before* you open any presentation software program [1–3].

## 3.1    Understanding Your Learners

First, you will need an understanding of who your learners are, and what they already know, in order to define the knowledge, attitudes, and skills you want them to be able to demonstrate by the end of your session. Ask a series of questions (of the learners themselves, or of a curriculum director) about previous exposure to the material, current level of mastery, and relative homogeneity or heterogeneity of the group. These questions are the first step in establishing "instructional empathy" – the ability to understand your learners and to see your presentation through their eyes. The answers to these questions will help you to define learning objectives for your particular audience (Fig. 3.1).

© The Author(s), under exclusive license to Springer Nature                    13
Switzerland AG 2021
E. P. Green, *Healthy Presentations*, https://doi.org/10.1007/978-3-030-72756-7_3

| Learners | Core Concepts | Teaching Strategies |
|---|---|---|
| **Who** are your learners?<br><br>**How** many are there?<br><br>**How** homogeneous or heterogeneous is the group?<br><br>**What** do they already know about the topic?<br><br>**How** does your session fit into the larger curriculum? | **What** are the main concepts you want your learners to take away?<br><br>**What** are the primary ideas you want them to understand?<br><br>**What** is the message you want them to hear? | **What** are the best teaching strategies for each of your main concepts?<br><br>**How** will you facilitate *active* learning? (see Chapter 4)<br><br>**How** will your learners demonstrate their knowledge? |

**Fig. 3.1**  Identifying learners, core concepts, and teaching strategies.

*Ask "who," "what," and "how" questions to better understand your learners and what they know. The answers to these questions will help you to define your presentation's core concepts, and choose appropriate teaching strategies.*

## 3.2   Defining Your Core Concepts

Next, you will need to think long and hard about the core concepts you want your learners to come away with. Not what you will "cover," but rather, what are the conceptual fundamentals of your talk? What are the concepts, theories, or ideas, which, if a learner fails to grasp, will make you feel as if the talk was a failure? These ideas form the foundation for your presentation, the core of what you will develop and deliver. They will define the scope of your content (Fig. 3.1).

Starting from a small set of learning outcomes and working in reverse toward your actual presentation is known as "backwards design," [6] and it places the appropriate emphasis on well-developed learning objectives. Worry less about your list of topics and more about what you want your learners to gain from your talk. All aspects of your presentation design (what you say, what you demonstrate, the activities you ask learners to engage in, etc.) should flow from the goals you set for your audience's learning.

> **Key Point**
> When crafting a talk, start with what you want your audience to learn, and work backward from there to achieve those outcomes.

The process of defining learning objectives is essential for curriculum development [6, 7]. On a macro level, programmatic objectives should drive the entire curriculum development process. Yet on the micro level, for individual presentations, the idea of "learning objectives" has become shorthand for yet another required slide at the beginning of every presentation. Often the slide is titled "Learning Objectives," but in fact it is a list of content areas the presenter plans to cover in his or her talk, or a list of objectives *for the lecture* ("We will then describe the different types of genetic malformations."), rather than *for the learners* ("At the end of this lecture learners will be able to describe the different types of genetic malformations."). As I mention later in this chapter, content outlines are very important, but they are fundamentally different from learning objectives.

## 3.3   Use of Active Verbs

When defining learning objectives, we get tripped up trying to use the ubiquitous list of cognitive action verbs generated from Bloom's taxonomy [4, 5]. We get so caught up in translating "I want them to understand…" to "They will be able to identify four main aspects of…" that we forget the real goals we set for our audience. While it is important to think about how learners might ultimately demonstrate the cognitive progress you want them to achieve (using specific, measurable verbiage such as "identify" or "describe"), in the early stages of presentation development it is important to keep things simple. Define informally, for yourself, your core concepts, and then design the talk around facilitating the understanding of those concepts. *What do you want your learners to learn, and how can you best facilitate that learning?*

> **Key Point**
> Do not worry about showing the list of learning objectives to your audience at the beginning of your talk. Despite current practices, objectives are "faculty-facing" as you develop your talk. Learners do not really need to see what it is they will be able to do post-lecture. Content outlines will be much more useful to learners in the moment.

When we do not engage in the important step of defining learning objectives and then work backward to design a talk that facilitates that learning, we tend to wander too far afield from our main ideas, or try to pack too much content into a single talk.

## 3.4   Identifying Appropriate Teaching Strategies

Finally, once you have defined appropriate objectives for your learners, you will need to give serious thought to how to facilitate that learning. Essentially, what are the best strategies, activities, or visual aids to use to help your learners build new knowledge (Fig. 3.1)? In Chap. 4, we will discuss teaching strategies you can incorporate into your presentations to facilitate "active" learning.

## 3.5   Beware the Inherited Slides

In medical education, there are often core lectures that do not change significantly from year to year. Basic physiology does not change, so why should the lecture slides? But occasionally the faculty member who traditionally gives a lecture has left the institution or is otherwise unavailable. So *you* have been asked to deliver the lecture. Given your new workload, having access to a previously developed slide deck can feel like a gift! However, *beware the inherited slide deck*.

It is essential that each presenter make their visual presentation their own. I recently had the experience of observing a presentation only to realize that it was the third time I had seen the slides, each time with a different presenter. The slides themselves were fine, but the delivery by the individuals who inherited the slides was problematic as it did not align with the information on the slides. The presenters skipped, or glossed over, content. There were awkward pauses as the presenter tried to figure out what a phrase meant, or why a particular diagram was included. The overall organization of content suffered as each presenter tried to fit his or her conceptual understanding of the material into someone else's framework. Using someone else's visuals had a negative impact on their own verbal delivery. (See Chap. 5 for more information about the anatomy of a presentation.)

> **Key Point**
> Do not attempt to deliver someone else's talk. Take the time to create your own presentation even if you have inherited a previously used slide deck.

If you inherit a slide deck, mine it for useful images including photographs, diagrams, and tables. Look for relevant citations and data that you may not have thought to include. Review the slides to make sure you understand the parameters of the talk, and to check that your content basically aligns with the content of the original presentation. However, I strongly encourage you to still engage in all of the lecture development steps and activities included in this chapter instead of defaulting to someone else's creation. Make the presentation your own in order to foster confidence in your content, and to ensure a smooth delivery.

The good news is that spending the time to understand your learners, to really think through what you want your learners to learn, and to develop appropriate teaching strategies, can help alleviate public speaking anxiety. The better we know our learners and our goals for those learners going into a presentation, the less likely that we will somehow stumble during the presentation delivery. We may even find that the teaching experience is more enjoyable and engaging for us as presenters.

The bad news of course is that all of this takes time. It takes time to craft a presentation based on learning goals, to design slides that support those goals, and even more time to practice our delivery. Yet if we truly value our roles as educators, if we are truly dedicated to the development of our learners and future colleagues, this is time well spent.

Once you have completed the steps above, it is (finally!) time to open up that software program and start crafting your presentation.

In biomedical education, presentations are often dense and complex. They are not the business world's streamlined stories of "visual persuasion" outlined in Cliff Atkinson's *Beyond Bullet Points* (2018). They do not lend themselves easily to formulaic outlines and rigid slide templates. Educational presentations are determined by some magical combination of learner needs, wondrous content, and presenter expertise. As educators, we create order and structure from that magical soup, delivering a cohesive narrative to our learners.

When we construct a talk, we should think about the entire scope of the narrative, with a beginning, middle, and end. We should pay particular attention to the transitions between parts – how we will begin, how we will maintain the audience's attention through the dense middle of our talk, and how we will wrap up our narrative at the end [1, 8].

## 3.6  Beginnings

We have a tendency to try and stick too many elements into the beginnings of talks. We introduce ourselves, show a title slide with our institutional affiliations, flash the ubiquitous disclaimer slide, read our learning objectives, and then review a detailed outline of the content we will be presenting. At that point, we are five minutes into the session and our audience has already settled in and taken out their phones. Any chance of grabbing their attention from the outset has passed us by.

I recommend that you craft the beginning of a talk with the following priorities: (1) introducing yourself as a means of orienting learners as to your positionality, and (2) launching as quickly as possible into a narrative "hook."

**Self-Introduction**  Introductions are often limited to name, title, and/or institutional affiliation. You should instead look at your self-introduction as an opportunity to orient learners as to the reason you are before them presenting this particular content. Why you? Why this? Introducing yourself is an opportunity to explain why you think they need to know the information you are about to teach [1].

"Positionality" refers to our socio-political identities and orientation as related to the content at hand. Identifying yourself as a clinician, clinical researcher, medical ethicist, or basic scientist, allows your audience to better understand your points of view.

Identifying myself as a white, cisgendered female educator may be a relevant portion of my own introduction, depending on the content and context of my presentation. Consider these two possible self-introductions for a presentation about this book:

> My name is Emily Green and I am the Assistant Dean for Faculty Development.

> My name is Emily Green. I'm here to talk with you today about a topic I am very passionate about. As an educator with almost two decades of experience watching and critiquing biomedical lectures, I believe that changes we make to the way we present can have an enormous impact on learning. I hope to have convinced you to begin making those changes by the time I finish today.

Which introduction gives me more credibility with the audience? Which creates a shared understanding of why I am in front of the audience that day?

**The Hook**  A "hook" is a narrative strategy to grab the attention of your learners at the outset of your talk [1, 8, 9]. Engagement is fundamental to learning – learners must be attending to you and to the information you are providing in order to construct new knowledge. Thus, it is imperative to think intentionally about how you will begin your presentation and grab learner attention early on.

An effective hook can take the form of a question, problem, case, or story. In Chap. 4, I talk in detail about the use of questions to facilitate active learning on the part of your audience. The key to using a question or a problem as a hook at the beginning of your presentation is that it not be rhetorical. After you briefly introduce yourself, pose the question or problem, and take a few moments to actively engage with learners before launching into additional content.

What kind of reaction is shown below? Is it from a first or second exposure, and how do you know?

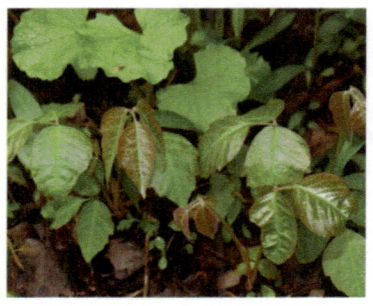 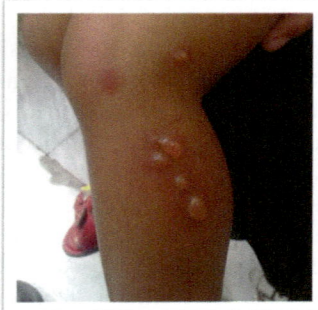

**Example 3.1** Using questions as a hook

*In this Example, the presenter uses questions and illustrative visuals to engage learners right away on the topic of hypersensitivity reactions. This slide could be the first or second slide in a presentation.*

A clinical case is a wonderful presentation hook. A case sends the message to learners that subsequent content has important clinical applications, which at least partially answers the audience question, "Why should I care?" Additionally, cases lend themselves to integration throughout a presentation. Grab their attention with the first part of the case, and then revisit the case throughout the talk as you gradually provide additional background and clinical information.

A case is one kind of story, but there are others you can use to get the attention of your audience. As human beings, we are hardwired for "plot" [1, 9–11]. We all love a good story. Consider beginning your presentation with a relevant, personal story about how you first engaged with the material, why you have dedicated your professional life to your field, or an experience you had the last time you presented this material.

**Key Point**
Rearranging portions of your talk into an unexpected sequence can be a way
to capture the attention of your audience.

Potential order:
1. Hook
2. Title slide and self-introduction
3. Presentation
4. Disclaimer statement (if no conflicts of interest to report)

Handouts/supplemental materials:
– Learning objectives
– References

**The Rest**  What about the rest of the slides that traditionally appear at the beginning
of a talk? Rearranging the title slide, disclaimer statement, learning objectives, and
content outline may be key to keeping your audience awake and engaged. Consider
putting your title slide *after* your hook. Ask the sponsoring office or department if
the required disclaimer slide can go at the *end* of your presentation (this would work
less well if you do in fact have disclaimers to make).

I mentioned above that properly written learning objectives should actually be
faculty-facing, not learner-facing. In other words, as you develop a talk the learning
objectives are for you – they should guide the development process. However, they
are fairly irrelevant to the learner experience *in the moment*. Ask if the list of learning objectives can be put at the end of your talk, or better yet in a handout (see Chap.
5 for the use and importance of handouts).

As for content outlines, I think they can be essential tools for orienting and reorienting your learners throughout a presentation. As such, I include them in the discussion below about constructing the "middles" of our talks.

## 3.7  Middles

Do you remember those photographs that were so popular a few years ago that
always featured a beautiful woman leading her handsome boyfriend by the hand
through their adventurous (and Instagram-perfect) life? Presenters are the Instagram

stars of their own talks! Presenters know the content of their talk better than anyone else at that moment, and as I mentioned in Chap. 2, it is their responsibility to lead the audience through the content [1, 12]. The more we hold learners' hands through difficult concepts and content transitions, the less they get lost or distracted, and the more efficient their learning. The more efficient their learning, the more swiftly and effectively they can build and retain new knowledge.

There are a number of ways to guide learners through the dense "middles" of our presentations.

**Parameters**  One way to lead your audience is to let them know ahead of time the parameters of your talk. "Today we are going to talk about X, we'll then explore a bit about Y, but I'm not going to spend too much time on Z." Parameters function like a really good title of an academic journal article – a good title very briefly elucidates the focus and scope of the research conducted.

By providing explicit parameters for your talk, you prime your learners for the content at hand – learners can begin tapping into any existing knowledge they may have on the topic, and get ready to build upon it [12, 13]. For example, when my kids and I were about to watch a televised performance of Hamilton, I did a quick mental survey to see what I could remember about the American founding fathers (not much as it turned out!) in order to prepare myself for the information to come.

Providing explicit parameters also prevents your audience from wasting important cognitive energy wondering what will and will not be covered in your talk. You can let them know the level of detail you will be discussing, and where they can go for additional information.

**Outline**  A second way to hold the hands of your learners is to use a content outline [12]. The key for outline use is that you revisit it repeatedly throughout the presentation. Often presenters review detailed outlines, with bullets and sub-bullets, at the beginning of their presentation. Once a presenter has read the second, possibly third topic that we will eventually get to hear about, they have lost me. I cannot "prime" my brain for each and every one of these topics, and I certainly cannot remember all of them for the entirety of the talk. So why go over the whole list at the outset? Instead, provide a brief sense of your talk's parameters (see above) and then use the outline as a way of orienting and reorienting your learners periodically throughout the talk to indicate what has been covered, and what is yet to come.

**Example 3.2**  Traditional content outline

**Example 3.3**  Traditional content outline, revised

*In addition to improvements in the background color and font style, Example 3.3 shows how an outline such as the one in Example 3.2 can be used as a reference point to orient and reorient learners. The presenter uses shapes, color, and text to indicate what has been covered so far and what is still to come.*

One benefit of using an outline this way, especially during very content-dense presentations, is that it prevents learners from cognitively wandering off for too long. At the next content transition, show the outline again and remind learners where you are in your narrative. That way they may have "lost" several minutes of your talk, but the whole hour (or whatever time remains) will not be wasted.

Outlines can also serve to orient *you* as the presenter. There is a tendency in scientific presentations to spend so much time on background information that presenters give short-shrift to the main concepts of their talk. Use an outline to remind yourself to proceed at a pace that will allow you to allocate adequate time to your main ideas!

An additional benefit of outline use is that it prevents learners from wasting precious cognitive energy wondering how much more content is going to be covered, and how much longer the talk will go on. In any presentation, whether as part of a course or at a professional conference, there is always some anxiety in the room as to whether or not you will adhere to a given schedule. Anything you can do to prevent that anxiety will decrease distraction, increase attention to the concepts at hand, and thus enhance learning.

One strategy to consider is including the number of slides per section as part of the outline (Example 3.4). This strategy makes explicit the relative "weight" of each section by indicating up front how many slides you are dedicating to each topic.

**Genome organization- Outline of topics for today**

- **DNA, Chromosome Structure** *(8 slides)*
- **Human Genome** *(5 slides)*
- **Gene structure, function** (Transcription, Translation, Regulation) *(8 slides)*
- **Classification of Genetic Disorders** *(3 slides)*
- **Sequencing changes** *(11 slides)*
    - Single nucleotide changes
    - Insertion
    - Deletion
    - Frameshift
    - Expanded repeats
- **Epigenetic changes** *(8 slides)*
- **Chromosomes, Cytogenetics** *(10 slides)*
    - Karyotype
    - Nomenclature
    - X-inactivation

**Example 3.4** Content outline with number of slides by section

*In this Example, the presenter includes the number of slides in each section of the session outline in an attempt to communicate relative length and weight of each section, and to decrease potential audience anxiety around seemingly "endless" slides.*

**Slide Numbers**  In general, I recommend against including slide numbers on your slides. For most presentations, they are unnecessary and act as a visual distraction. However, for very brief presentations, of twenty minutes or less perhaps, slide numbers that indicate progression out of the total number of slides can serve to decrease the "schedule anxiety" I mentioned above.

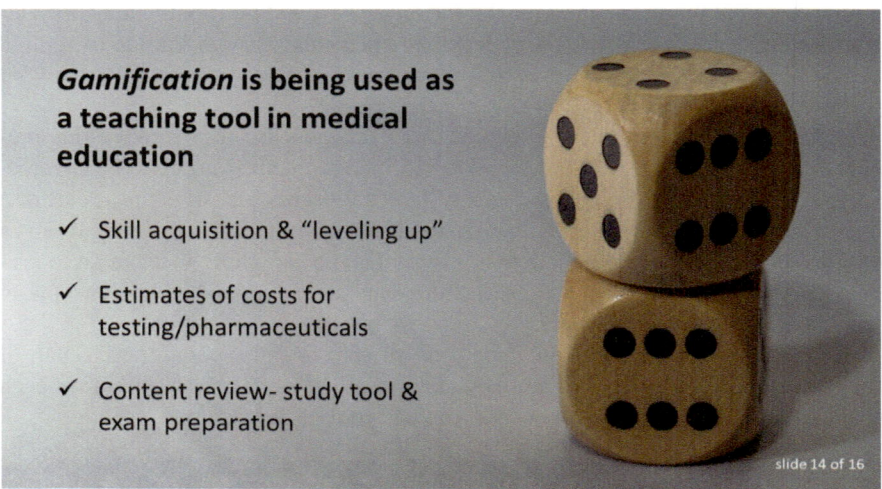

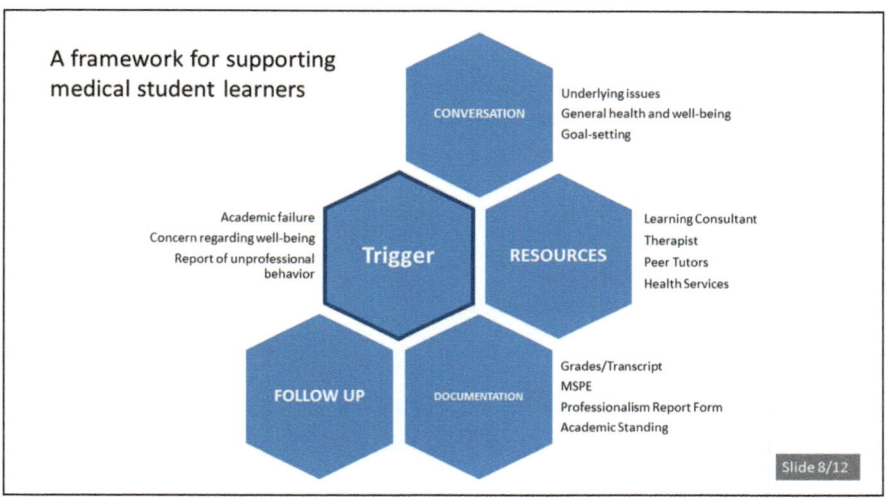

**Examples 3.5 & 3.6**  Use of slide numbers, option 1 and 2

*In the Examples here, learners are reassured that the total number of slides is low, and that the presenter is nearing the end of his or her presentation. The audience can focus on the topic at hand rather than worrying about the session getting off-schedule.*

## 3.8  Endings

It is always so disappointing when a good talk ends abruptly, either because the presenter has run out of time, or because the presenter fails to cue the audience that he or she is wrapping up. When a presenter goes straight from content-explanation to a "thank you" or acknowledgments slide, the audience becomes disoriented, and more importantly, an opportunity to facilitate content retention is lost [1].

We facilitate *comprehension* when the organization of content is logical, when transitions are seamless, and when we reduce as much as possible all distractions from the core concepts we have identified. We facilitate *retention* of that material when we review and reinforce our main concepts. Do not waste the opportunity to strategically use your final slides to review and reinforce your main ideas. End your presentation with a handful of "pearls," "tips," or main takeaway messages from your talk. Use your final slides to summarize content, or detail the conclusions you want your learners to draw from the material you have presented.

Once you have provided a summary or otherwise concluded your content presentation, you can then move on to ask if there are any questions, thank relevant individuals, provide your contact information, or show a reference list (see Chap. 5 for additional information about appropriate ways to provide references). Other ways to end your talk include asking your audience to commit to a particular action or behavior change (see Chap. 4 for a discussion of commitment as a teaching tool), presenting a final mini-quiz or assignment (see Chap. 4 for examples), or asking your audience to reflect, either out loud or in writing, on what they learned.

The content of a *healthy presentation* is appropriately targeted to the audience, designed to advance specific learning objectives, and conveyed in a way that facilitates comprehension and retention. "Hook" your learners early on, and then hold their hands as you lead them through the core concepts of your talk. Crafting a *healthy presentation* requires what I call "instructional empathy" – a process of putting yourself in your learners' shoes. Try to see your presentation through their eyes. Does it meet your needs? Does it keep you engaged? *Does it advance your learning?* No presentation is perfect. No presenter is perfect. Yet we can all do a better job of making sure that our presentations are teacher-delivered, yet learner-centered.

**Summary Points**
- There are a number of steps to take *before* you open any presentation software programs and start designing your slides.
- Taking steps to understand who your learners are, and what they already know, will help you target your presentation appropriately.
- Identify what you want your audience to learn, and the teaching strategies that will best facilitate that learning.

- Mine any inherited slide decks for key content, but be sure to make the presentation your own.
- "Hook" the audience's attention early on, and reorient them periodically as you move through your content.
- Use your final slides to reinforce your main concepts.

## References

1. Alley M. The craft of scientific presentations: critical steps to succeed and critical errors to avoid. 2nd ed. New York: Springer; 2013.
2. Nathans-Kelly T, Nicometo CG. Slide rules: design, build, and archive presentations in the engineering and technical fields, vol. 3. Hoboken: Wiley; 2014.
3. Reynolds G. Presentation Zen design: a simple visual approach to presenting in today's world. Berkeley: Pearson Education; 2014.
4. Anderson LW, Bloom BS. A taxonomy for learning, teaching, and assessing: a revision of Bloom's taxonomy of educational objectives. New York: Longman; 2001.
5. Bloom BS. Taxonomy of educational objectives: the classification of educational goals. Handbook 1: cognitive domain. New York: David McKay Co. Inc.; 1956.
6. Wiggins GP, McTighe J. Understanding by design. Alexandria: Association for Supervision and Curriculum Development; 1998.
7. Thomas PA, Kern DE, Hughes MT, Chen BY, editors. Curriculum development for medical education: a six-step approach. Baltimore: JHU Press; 2016.
8. Atkinson C. Beyond bullet points: using Microsoft PowerPoint to create presentations that inform, motivate, and inspire (Bpg-other). Microsoft Press; 2005.
9. Easton G. How medical teachers use narratives in lectures: a qualitative study. BMC Med Educ. 2016;16(1):3.
10. Bruner J. Life as narrative. Soc Res: An International Quarterly. 2004;71(3):691–710.
11. Rossiter M. Understanding adult development as narrative. New Dir Adult Contin Educ. 1999;1999(84):77–85.
12. Mayer RE. Multimedia learning. Cambridge: Cambridge University Press; 2009.
13. Lang JM. Small teaching: everyday lessons from the science of learning. San Francisco: Wiley; 2016.

# Chapter 4
# Incorporating Opportunities for Active Learning

**Abstract**
This chapter makes the case that because our goal is the facilitation of learning, we should integrate teaching strategies into our presentations that encourage students to actively engage with our content, even if these activities use some portion of our allotted time. Intentional use of questioning is the most familiar and efficient way to facilitate active learning. Other strategies include the use of "workshop" activities, mini-assignments, and branching-plot cases. *Healthy presentations* require learners to engage in an array of cognitive processes, help learners build upon prior knowledge, and facilitate the retention of content.

The goal of all teaching should be to facilitate "active" learning on the part of our audience. Thus, every presentation should incorporate teaching strategies designed to help meet that goal.

## 4.1 Defining Active Learning

In some ways, it is easier to define active learning by what it is not. It is *not* passive absorption of information, as if through osmosis. It is *not* a "sage on the stage," and an audience full of empty vessels waiting to be filled with wisdom. We know now that learning does not happen this way [1–6].

Teaching that facilitates active learning is teaching that asks learners to engage in an array of cognitive processes to help build upon prior knowledge [5, 7–11]. Through these cognitive processes – such as identifying, defining, classifying, comparing and contrasting, prioritizing, criticizing, reframing, applying, creating, and so on – learners expand their understanding, and build new knowledge.

E. P. Green, *Healthy Presentations*, https://doi.org/10.1007/978-3-030-72756-7_4

Active cognition verbs should be familiar to all of us from Bloom's taxonomy of thinking skills [12, 13]. They should also be familiar to anyone who has done any curriculum development that involves the writing of learning objectives – these are the verbs we are asked to use to complete the sentence, "At the end of this activity, learners will be able to…"

Building opportunities for active learning into lectures, which have traditionally been a teaching modality that encourages passive participation (notice that I do not use the term "passive learning" as little learning happens when passivity characterizes the interaction), can be a challenge. Yet many of the strategies I mention below are relatively easy to implement.

## 4.2  Use of Questions

Strategic use of questions is the most efficient way to facilitate engagement and active learning within a lecture. It is also the most familiar to faculty. Integrating questions into your lecture can be as easy as asking, "What is this?" or "What do you see?" every time you put up a slide that contains a picture, diagram, photograph, or table, rather than launching automatically into your *own* explanation.

The real goal of questioning is to get as many people in the room as possible to cognitively "chew" on the question posed, and then on the basis of that cognitive processing, to commit to a particular answer.

> **Key Point**
> Use questions to cognitively engage as many learners as possible.

**Transform "Q & A" to "Q W & A"**  Often, when we pose a question to the audience of our lecture, we experience anxiety that no one will raise their hand. We are so concerned about preventing awkwardness, and so uncomfortable with silence, that we pounce on the first hand that we see go up in the air. At that point, the Q & A process is unfortunately a 1:1 interaction. We only know for sure that a single learner is actively processing our question, and by calling on that learner so quickly, other learners may stop trying to answer the question on their own, and are now simply waiting to see what the "right" answer is.

One way to get more people in the room engaged in answering a question is to add a "W" (Wait) to the Q & A process. "QW & A" does not roll off the tongue nearly as easily as "Q & A" does, but it is an easy and effective strategy.

The next time you pose a question to your audience, wait ("W"). If you are uncomfortable you can fill the silence by indicating, "Let's see if we can get some additional hands up," or "I see one hand up, how about some others?" Only then do you call on someone to answer, and either agree and expand on their answer, or correct and explain why it was inaccurate. In this way, your 1:1 interaction hopefully becomes a 1:5 or 1:10 or even 1:30 interaction, with additional learners engaged in trying to answer your question.

You could potentially also break this down into a three-step process.

1. First, pose the question.
2. Second, ask for a show of hands of learners who have an answer in mind ("Hands up if you think you know the answer, or have an answer you *think* might be right.").
3. Third, ask them to keep their hands raised if they are willing to share their answer. This way you have encouraged cognitive participation and commitment from *all* learners, even if ultimately only one learner verbally shares his or her answer.

**Transform "Q & A" to "Q D & A"**   In a similar way, we can expand the number of engaged learners when a question comes to us from the audience. Our first instinct may be to launch into an answer. After all, that is why we are up here, to teach! But how many more learners might you engage if you deflected ("D") the question instead, at least initially? "Great question, what do you all think?" "Anyone else want to take a stab at answering that?" Then, as before, you can either agree and expand, or correct and explain.

Adding Wait and Deflect to our usual Q & A takes practice, but they are relatively simple ways of increasing the portion of your audience engaged in active learning.

**Audience Response**   The use of audience response systems as part of the Q & A process is relatively common in medical education these days. Phone or device-based systems are effective in increasing even further the number of learners who attempt to answer your question.

The most effective use of audience response I have witnessed was at the Association for Medical Education in Europe's (AMEE) 2019 international conference on faculty development in the health professions. The facilitators posed an opinion question to the general session about whether or not we thought medical faculty should have mandatory training on how to teach. They then staged a debate where one presenter presented an argument in the affirmative, and one in the negative. After a chance for rebuttal, the session facilitators released the same question again, to see how the audience's opinion had been changed or reinforced by the two presentations. The presenter who changed the most people's minds "won" the debate.

Let us think for a moment about what the facilitators asked of us through the use of the audience response system. The question posed ("Should medical educators have to engage in mandatory training on how to teach?") was relevant to all of the earlier workshops in which we had been participating for the past several days. As such, it built upon our previous knowledge of the topic at hand. In order to answer the question, we needed to (1) review information gained previously, (2) critique the options presented, (3) prioritize one over the other, and (4) commit to an answer.

> **Key Point**
> Asking learners to commit to an answer requires that they cognitively engage with the content at hand.

*Commitment is the hallmark of audience response as a teaching strategy.* By presenting a limited number of options and asking your learners to commit to one of them, you are facilitating the active cognitive processes that precede it. The processes of reviewing, critiquing, and prioritizing, all inform and allow the audience members' commitment.

Presenting poll results publicly allows your learners to review their answer relative to how others answered, or in the case of the conference I mentioned, to evaluate the success of pro and con arguments.

Not all audience response needs to involve devices or software. Low-tech options, such as having learners raise their hands, hold up colored "voting" cards, or stand up to indicate agreement or disagreement, are also easy-to-implement teaching strategies.

In Chap. 8, I discuss the use of audience response in virtual teaching.

**Turn and Talk** Sometimes learners would benefit from being able to discuss a question with a partner before committing to an answer. In these cases, you can facilitate a brief "turn and talk" activity. Simply pose the question or problem, then have your learners turn to the person next to them to discuss it and come up with an answer together.

One version of a "turn and talk" is "think, pair, share," in which learners take a moment to think, and perhaps write, on their own, before discussing those thoughts with a partner. In both of these cases, pairs can then share their thinking with the larger group.

## 4.3   Workshop Elements

We tend to classify truly interactive sessions as "workshops" rather than "presentations." Yet perhaps, we should be incorporating simple workshop elements into more of our traditional lectures to better facilitate active learning and engagement with the material. If indeed the default settings of presentation software are too constraining in their encouragement of unidirectional information transfer (see Chap. 5 for more information), we should integrate other elements into our presentations that widen our range of potential teaching strategies and practices, and free ourselves from the traditional didactic "enactment" of slide decks [14].

> **Key Point**
> Incorporating quick, interactive elements into traditional lectures may help facilitate learning.

Workshop elements do not have to take a great deal of time, but again, remember that the goal of our presentations is not to "cover" material. The goal of every lecture is to facilitate learning [15]. To that end, if brief activities help learners engage with the material and to build new knowledge, we should not worry about diverting a few minutes away from content "delivery" to interactive elements.

**Role play**   The use of role play in medical education ranges from complex simulations in specialized environments ("sim centers"), to simple interactions with standardized patients, or even brief scripted interactions between peers. The use of role play within a traditional lecture can be even more straightforward, and can be particularly useful in presentations regarding communication skills, such as having difficult conversations, delivering bad news, or calling out mistreatment or bias.

> Let us use a presentation to second-year medical students on motivational interviewing as an example. The presenter has been talking about self-efficacy, and how to help patients identify strategies they have used successfully in the past. The presenter then asks for volunteers – "What exactly would you say to the patient to help them identify positive coping strategies? Pretend I'm the patient, what words would you use?"
>
> Asking learners to verbally articulate their thinking in role play form, rather than simply describe their thoughts hypothetically, is a form of experiential learning. The volunteer(s) get to experience how difficult it is to put delicate thoughts into words, the importance of tone, and how easy it is to stumble or reveal nervousness. This kind of role play is very brief, and admittedly involves a very limited number of learners, but with appropriate debriefing afterward, can be a powerful teaching tool, especially for learners who may otherwise struggle with appropriate word choice or phrasing.

**Fishbowl**   A fishbowl exercise is one in which the audience is arranged into two layers – the small inner layer of two-to-four individuals who actively engage in a discussion, debate, or problem-solving process, and the rest of the audience who observes the inner layer as if they were in a "fishbowl." Within a fairly quick time frame, and with some planning at the outset, a presenter can ask for a small number of volunteers to come to the front of the lecture hall (or middle of the room), as the rest of the audience observes.

> Let us use a resident noon conference on headache as an example. The presenter has been discussing the case of an adolescent girl with autism who presents with persistent headache symptoms. The presenter asks two volunteers to come forward and discuss differential diagnoses and appropriate imaging, and to talk through the management of the conversation with the patient's family. The rest of the audience listens to their discussion and reasoning, and, after a few minutes, debriefs as a large group.

**Opinion Spectrum** An opinion spectrum is a nuanced variation of audience response. Rather than asking learners to choose an answer from a small number of predetermined choices, an opinion spectrum allows learners to physically demonstrate a choice along a continuum.

> For example, in the conference debate example I mentioned previously, the session facilitators could have indicated that one side of the room represented "strong agreement" that medical educators should undergo mandated training in teaching. The opposite side of the room could have represented "strong disagreement" with that notion. They could then ask participants to physically move to a location that represented their opinion along that agreement continuum.
>
> After the debate, participants could move to a new location that represented their updated opinions. An opinion spectrum is a physical demonstration of the kind of commitment, and preceding cognitive processes, mentioned earlier in this chapter.

## 4.4   Mini-Assignments

It is perhaps a regrettable truth that assessment can drive learning. When the content you present is relevant to an upcoming exam or assessment, learners have an additional, if extrinsic, motivation to engage with the material. However, even when your presentation is not directly tied to an assessment, it is possible to increase learner engagement through the use of mini-assignments. *These assignments do not themselves necessarily facilitate deep learning, but knowledge of assignments ahead of time may increase learner attention and motivation to engage in the moment.*

> **Key Point**
> If learners know about an assignment ahead of time, they may be motivated to stay engaged in the presentation.

**Quick-Write** Give your learners one minute to write down as many facts as they can remember from your talk. Also sometimes called a one-minute paper, this brief writing assignment can also be done prior to a talk ("Write down everything you know about today's topic.") to activate learners' relevant knowledge and get them engaged.

**Haiku**  Have your learners create a three-line (5 syllables, 7 syllables, 5 syllables) poem that captures one of the main concepts you covered in your talk.

> **An Active Learning Haiku**
> *Activate their brains*
> *Use questions; think, pair and share*
> *They will remember*

**Summary Tweet**  Have your learners summarize your presentation in 280 characters. You can then share these "tweets" with the group.

**3-Question Quiz**  Ask your learners to write three review questions (with answers) from your presentation. You can then compile and distribute the questions to the whole group.

**2 Truths and a Lie**  Ask your learners to write down three facts from your presentation, only two of which are true. They should also include a rationale for why the one fact is not actually "fact." You can then compile and distribute the facts to the whole group for discussion or out-of-class review.

## 4.5   Case-Based Learning

As mentioned in Chap. 3, the use of clinical cases can be a powerful tool to engage your audience, and to alert them to relevant clinical applications of your content. While wonderful tools to encourage discussion, case studies unfortunately tend to unfold with a singular plot, predetermined by the presenter.

One way to engage your audience is to build decision points into your cases that lead to branching plot lines. Much like Edward Packard's *Choose Your Own Adventure* stories that were so popular with children in the 1980s, this type of case allows your learners to evaluate their options, choose a course of action, and identify the consequences of that choice, without any risk.

For example, in a presentation about pain management, a presenter could include a case about a patient recently diagnosed with advanced lung cancer (Example 4.1). The presenter asks the audience to evaluate the safety of sending the patient home with high-dose opioids given a history of depression, and to choose between two possible courses of action. Most presentation software programs include the ability to insert hyperlinks into text or shapes. Those hyperlinks will take you to a different slide within the same presentation, depending on the audience's choice, thus allowing the case to unfold across a variety of possible scenarios with a simple click of the mouse.

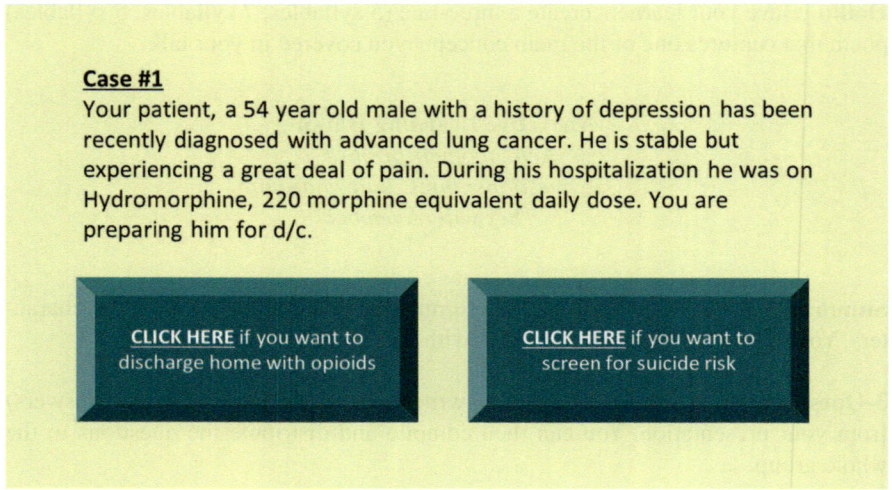

**Example 4.1**  Branching-plot clinical case

*In this Example, the presenter engages the learners by asking them to commit to a course of action. The case can proceed in two different directions through links to different slides within the same slide deck.*

For example, if the learners choose to prioritize pain management via opioids, the presenter can click on a link to a slide that shows the potential consequences of doing so, and the case proceeds. If the learners choose to screen the patient for suicide risk, the presenter clicks on that option, and proceeds to a different slide. A branching-plot case design does take additional work to set up. However, it is an additional means to engage your learners and have them actively engage with the material.

The definition of good teaching is the facilitation of (active) learning. While lectures tend to have the bad reputation of enabling passivity on the part of our learners, it is possible to facilitate active learning in all kinds of teaching, especially in *healthy presentations*. In Chap. 8, I discuss how you can integrate opportunities for active learning into virtual presentations as well.

**Summary Points**
- Presentations can and should involve opportunities for active learning on the part of participants.
- When you pose a question, wait for multiple raised hands before you call on someone, in order to engage as many learners as possible.
- When a question is posed to you from the audience, deflect it to other learners before answering, in order to engage as many learners as possible.

- High- and low-tech audience response systems encourage learners to "commit" to a question's answer.
- Integrate various "workshop" elements into your presentations to facilitate active learning.

# References

1. Barr RB, Tagg J. From teaching to learning—a new paradigm for undergraduate education. Change: The Magazine of Higher Learning. 1995;27(6):12–26.
2. Brown PC, Roediger HL III, McDaniel MA. Make it stick. Harvard University Press; 2014.
3. Dunlosky J, Rawson KA, Marsh EJ, Nathan MJ, Willingham DT. Improving students' learning with effective learning techniques: promising directions from cognitive and educational psychology. Psychol Sci Public Interest. 2013;14(1):4–58.
4. Lang JM. Small teaching: everyday lessons from the science of learning. San Francisco: Wiley; 2016.
5. Mayer RE. Multimedia learning. Cambridge, Cambridge University Press; 2009.
6. Merriam SB, Caffarella R, Baumgartner S. Learning in adulthood: A comprehensive guide. 3rd ed. San Francisco: Jossey-Bass; 2007.
7. Fornari A, Poznanski A, editors. How-to guide for active learning. International Association of Medical Science Educators. Springer Nature Switzerland.
8. Michael J. Where's the evidence that active learning works? Adv Physiol Educ. 2006;30:159.
9. Prince M. Does active learning work? A review of the research. J Eng Educ. 2004;93(3):223–31.
10. Rideout M, Held M, Holmes AV. The didactic makeover: keep it short, active, relevant. Pediatrics. 2016;138(1):e20160751.
11. Wolff M, Wagner MJ, Poznanski S, Schiller J, Santen S. Not another boring lecture: engaging learners with active learning techniques. J Emerg Med. 2015;48(1):85–93.
12. Anderson LW, Bloom BS. A taxonomy for learning, teaching, and assessing: a revision of Bloom's taxonomy of educational objectives. New York: Longman; 2001.
13. Bloom BS. Taxonomy of educational objectives: the classification of educational goals. Handbook 1: cognitive domain. New York: David McKay Co. Inc.; 1956.
14. Kernbach S, Bresciani S. 10 years after Tufte's" cognitive style of PowerPoint": synthesizing its constraining qualities. In: 2013 17th international conference on information visualisation. IEEE; 2013, July. p. 345–50.
15. Wiggins GP, McTighe J. Understanding by design. Alexandria: Association for Supervision and Curriculum Development; 1998.

# Chapter 5
# The Basics of Slide Design

**Abstract**

This chapter describes the three components that make up the anatomy of a presentation, and the use of supplemental materials to reduce reliance on text-based slides. It reviews the "assertion-evidence" approach to slide design, and provides five general rules to guide the design of biomedical slides. These rules include the following: (1) Find opportunities to use text differently. (2) Simple is better. (3) Visual elements should be relevant and informative. (4) Text and visual elements should be large and readable. (5) Your slides should include color, space, and a variety of images. Simple changes, such as using visual elements instead of bulleted lists, can transform our conventional presentations into *healthy presentations*.

Before we delve into the particulars of good slide design, we need to consider the anatomy of a presentation. Our slides do not exist in isolation [1]. They represent one of three components that make up our teaching. Learners access all three of these components to increase their understanding of the content at hand.

## 5.1 Anatomy of a Presentation

In their book, *Slide Rules*, Nathans-Kelly and Nicometo (2014) talk about the two lives of a presentation – one in the moment of delivery, the other as an archive. I would argue that the complete anatomy of a presentation consists of (1) the verbal delivery (what you say), (2) the visual delivery (what you show), and (3) any and all supplemental materials (what you provide) (Fig. 5.1).

Importantly, the way in which we design our verbal delivery and supplemental materials can and should influence how we design our slides. (See Chap. 7 for a discussion on the verbal delivery portion of presentations.) In other words, the three components of

E. P. Green, *Healthy Presentations*, https://doi.org/10.1007/978-3-030-72756-7_5

**Fig. 5.1** Anatomy of a
presentation

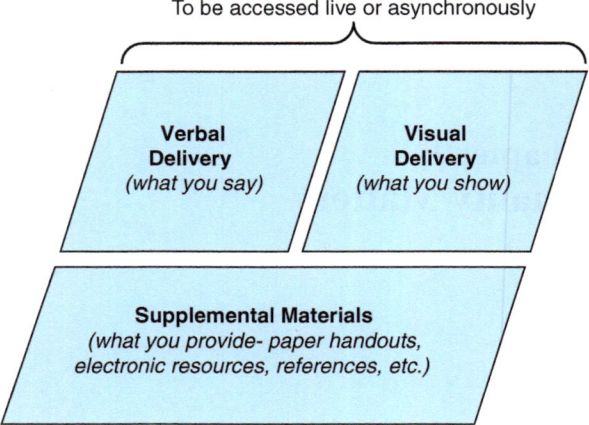

a presentation do not exist in isolation. What we plan to say, and what we plan to provide, will impact our slide design plan. Each of these plans should be executed to support the specific learning objectives you identified for your presentation (see Chap. 3).

**Supplemental Materials** As you develop your presentation and make decisions about the core concepts you want your audience to learn, you should ask yourself if particular content is best be delivered verbally, on a slide, or within some kind of supplemental material [2]. Not everything is appropriate to put on your slides, and *the more you deliver in supplemental form, the cleaner and less text-heavy your slides.*

> IF content is core to what you want your audience to learn, THEN it belongs in your verbal delivery, your visual delivery, or both.
>
> IF content is highly detailed, potentially tangential, primarily useful for exam preparation, or otherwise needed for reference at a later date, THEN consider taking it out of your slides (visual delivery) and putting it in a handout or electronic resource (supplemental materials).

Supplemental materials can be in paper form as handouts, in electronic form, or both. Common supplemental materials include the following:

- Copies of presentation slides
- Copies of presentation slides with presenter notes
- Presenter notes
- Extension material with additional relevant details
- Review questions
- Exam preparatory material
- References
- Academic articles
- Databases
- Archived content housed on a learning management system (LMS) such as Canvas, Blackboard, or another website
- Shared learner-created notes

In college courses, and even in undergraduate medical education courses, we can reasonably expect that learners are taking notes during presentations, and that these notes act as a sort of lecture archive. But we tend not to have this expectation when it comes to presentations in front of residents or our peers, or in contexts such as professional conferences. In these instances, the onus is on us to create materials that extend learners' understanding, provide additional detail, and that learners can access asynchronously *after* a presentation.

The most important part of a presentation is *you*. Your slides play a supporting role. Your supplemental materials play an even more supporting role. Let them carry some of the weight of your content. Let learners access supplemental materials on their own time after your presentation, as many times as they need. Use this third component of your presentation as an enduring product to help facilitate learning asynchronously.

> **Key Point**
> Good design becomes so much easier when we take away the pressure to dump everything onto our slides.

*"Your slides are too wordy."*

When I die, I think this phrase is going to go on my headstone. It can be said of almost every presentation I have ever seen, and many of the ones that I have given myself. It is a ubiquitous problem, but the fact is, even when we recognize that our slides are too wordy, it can be hard to figure out how exactly to change them.

## 5.2   Common Slide Design

The myriad of issues with the default settings of slide presentation software are well documented [1–6]. Settings that consist of a heading followed by lists of bullets and sub-bullets lead to text-heavy slides. We need to learn to use text differently. *Rather than acting as cue cards to stimulate every word of our verbal delivery, text should be used to strategically support audience learning.*

For example, a very common slide design consists of a series of bulleted text on the left and a graph or visual element on the right (Example 5.1) [2, 3]. This arrangement would seem to align with the tenets of multimedia instruction laid out in Mayer's book, *Multimedia Learning* (2009). Multimedia instruction is the use of both words and pictures in such a way that learners create connections between the two. Mayer's principle of spatial contiguity indicates that words and pictures should be arranged near to one another in physical space to reduce the "cognitive load" required of learners who need to switch back and forth between the two sources of information [7]. However in reality, this particular slide design, while a favorite of presenters everywhere, is an example of an over-reliance on a generic bulleted list, and a visual aid that is too small to be read easily. The fact that words and an image are next to each other is secondary to the other problems with this particular slide design.

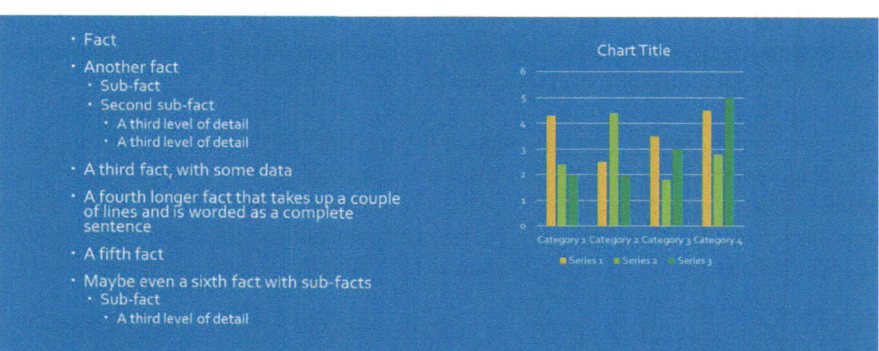

**Example 5.1**   Traditional slide design with bulleted text and image

*A common slide design is one that includes a vague heading and a bulleted text-based list next to a relevant visual image or graph.*

While a presenter may spend significant time verbally explaining the information illustrated by graphs on slides like Example 5.1, frequently the written text does little to make clear the appropriate conclusions to be drawn by the audience [3, 7]. The text tends to be descriptive, but not instructive. "The cognitive processes involved in sense-making can be facilitated by a clear and concise summary" (Mayer, 2009, p. 103). In other words, help facilitate learning by clearly explicating what you want learners to take away from each slide.

Audience learning of the information presented in Example 5.1 might be better facilitated if the presenter (1) made the graph bigger, (2) relocated any sub-level details of the bulleted list to the supplemental materials component of the presentation, and (3) used group discussion to answer the questions, "What does this graph tell us?" "What conclusions can we come to based on this data?" "Why is this data important?" The presenter could then include the answers to these questions on a summary slide, or in an "assertion" as the heading of a slide.

## 5.3   Assertion-Evidence Design

In his book, *The Craft of Scientific Presentations: Critical Steps to Succeed and Critical Errors to Avoid* (2013), Michael Alley promotes what he calls the "assertion-evidence" approach to slide design. Using this format, the presenter provides an assertion in the form of a complete sentence in the top left corner of the slide. The assertion represents the conclusion the presenter would like the audience to draw. Visual evidence that supports the presenter's assertion is included in the body of the slide. Text is used to instruct, and visuals are used to support that instruction. According to studies conducted by Alley and colleagues on the assertion-evidence approach, learners better understood and retained information when complex content was presented in this format [8, 9].

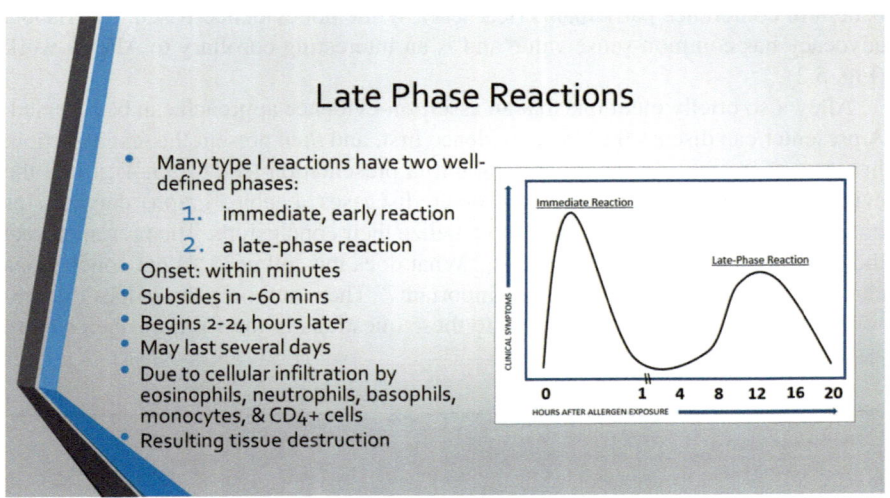

**Example 5.2**  Traditional slide design using default settings

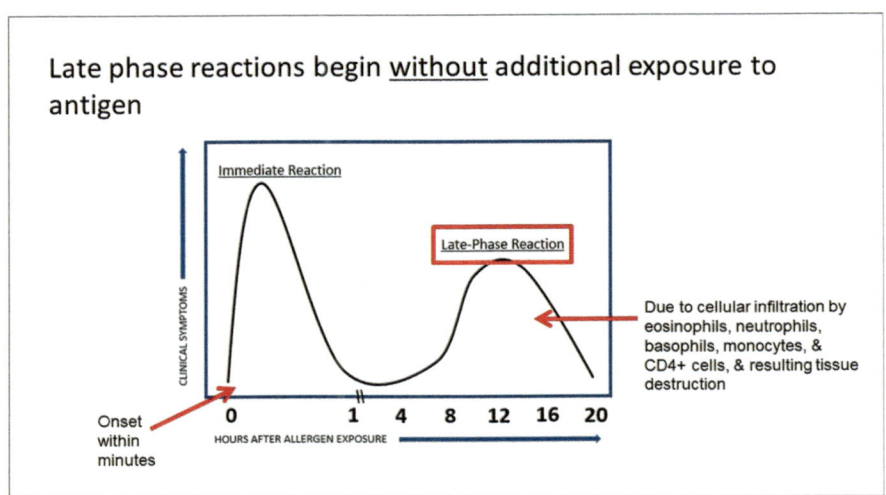

**Example 5.3**  Assertion-evidence slide design

*Example 5.3 is an example of "assertion-evidence" slide design. Example 5.2 has been revised such that the salient clinical issue (the fact that late-phase reactions happen without additional exposure to the initial antigen) is highlighted as an "assertion" at the top of the slide to help promote learner retention of important conclusions.*

A new approach to academic poster design, spearheaded by Mike Morrison in his popular video, "How to create a better research poster in less time" (2019) [10], seems aligned with Alley's vision for presentations. Morrison advocates for poster design that is both conceptually and spatially centered around a main assertion. All other information is relegated to supporting positions along the poster's periphery. According to Morrison, this design provides maximum experiential and educational benefit to conference participants (learners). While not evidence-based, Morrison's advocacy has common-sense value and is an interesting corollary to Alley's work (Fig. 5.2).

Alley also briefly mentions that an assertion-evidence approach can be reversed. A presenter can discuss the visual evidence first, and *then* present the text assertion. In terms of integrating active learning into a presentation (see Chap. 4), I like the evidence-assertion approach. A presenter discusses a table, graph, diagram, or image, and then asks the audience to verbalize their conclusions. The presenter asks the *audience* to answer the questions, "What does this tell us?" "What conclusions can we come to?" and "Why is this important?" Then, and only then, does the presenter show his or her own answers to these questions in the form of one or more assertions.

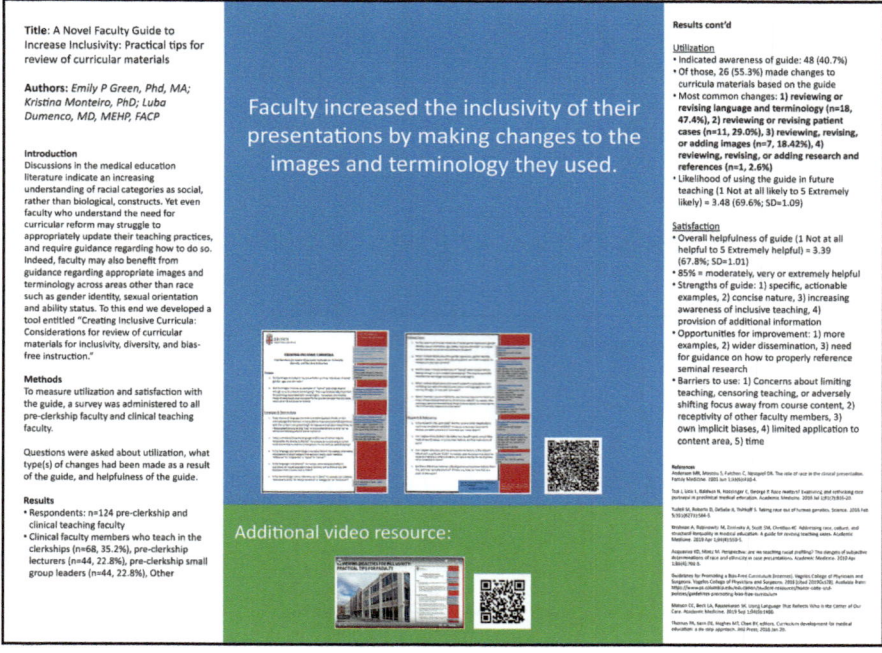

**Fig. 5.2** Academic poster design using assertion-evidence principle

*As you can see in this image of an academic poster created using Morrison's suggested poster design, the main finding of the study (the "assertion") is large, centrally positioned, and succinctly stated. The details of the study and references are included, but positioned along the sides of the poster.*

Of course, not all content is amenable to the assertion-evidence (or evidence-assertion) approach to slide design. In medicine and the biomedical sciences, dense slides are a necessity, and the information to be conveyed may not lend itself conceptually to singular images and assertions. The perfect supporting image, whether it be a photograph, table, or graph, does not always exist.

Below are five general rules to help guide your slide design for biomedical presentations.

Rule #1: *Find opportunities to use text differently*

Once you have determined that your content requires a text-based slide, there may still be ways to design it that promote visual interest, and that actually enhance the content via the visual illustration of an abstract concept [11]. In her 2008 book *Slide:ology*, Nancy Duarte includes an array of diagrams used to communicate abstract concepts such as relative importance, cohesion, separation, emphasis, cause and effect, and process. Many of these diagrams are very simple, and creating them involves strategic use of color and of basic tools embedded in PowerPoint, Google Slides, and other presentation software, such as insertion of shapes and PowerPoint's "SmartArt" [1].

Again, the goal is not to get rid of *all* text, the goal is to identify appropriate opportunities to present text-based information in ways that (1) engage learner attention by breaking up the procession of visually similar slides, and (2) facilitate increased comprehension and retention of complex information. Below I highlight a number of opportunities to impart information common to medical presentations using visual depictions.

Opportunities to use text differently include the following:

- Bulleted lists
- Timelines and stages
- Geographical concepts
- Visual metaphors

**The Bulleted List**   The use of bulleted lists is ubiquitous in medical and scientific presentations. Unfortunately, bulleted lists do not allow for easy prioritization of one piece of information over another, do not indicate what is *excluded* from a list, and do not easily illustrate relationships between pieces of information [4, 6, 7]. Conceptual ideas of importance, size, cause and effect, and connection are all poorly communicated when bulleted facts and sentence fragments are the design default.

A learning specialist told Ginny, the hypothetical medical student we met in Chap. 1, that she was having difficulty "seeing the forest through the trees." This is a common problem when a learner encounters list after list of bulleted information. Those core concepts that you outlined when you began to craft your presentation (Chap.3), the main ideas you wanted your audience to learn, can easily get lost [7, 12, 13]. *We present so many bulleted "trees" that our audience loses sight of the conceptual forest.* "Seeing the whole of something – the forest rather than the trees, the image of the newspaper photo rather than its dots – gives meaning to its elements, and that whole becomes more than a sum of component parts" (Barr & Tagg, 1995, p. 21).

Traditional text-based slides rely heavily on lists of information that are vertical in design, and that unfold in a linear fashion. The audience is expected to start at the top and visually work their way downward, each bullet followed by another. We are so used to this progression, that it feels "natural." As presenters, it does not occur to us that alternate designs could provide visual respite from the norm, and potentially communicate more and better information.

In order to help learners better understand the relationship between pieces of information, consider putting content that is of equal importance into colored

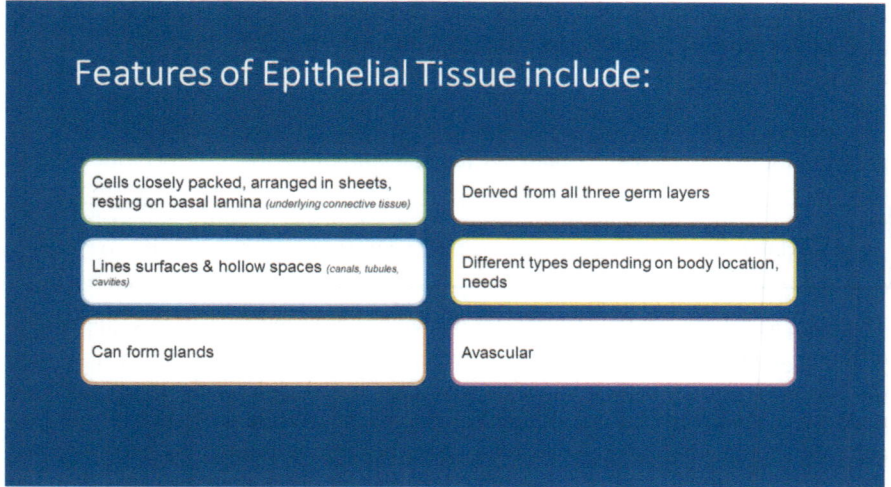

**Example 5.4**  Traditional bulleted list

**Example 5.5**  Traditional bulleted list, revised using shapes

*The vertically arranged bulleted list of Example 5.4 has been revised in Example 5.5 as a visual "array" of content elements that are conceptually linked and of equal importance.*

shapes. This type of slide design is very similar in nature to a bulleted list of text, but the addition of color and shapes provides additional visual interest, and more importantly serves to illustrate in an *intentional* way, *membership*, *relative equity*, and *separation* (Example 5.5).

You can transform your list of bulleted text into equal portions of a large shape to indicate *membership in a larger cohesive whole* (Example 5.7), or into a cluster of shapes for content that includes areas of conceptual overlap or linkage. You can also utilize horizontally arranged text and shapes to illustrate membership, hierarchy, and categorization (Example 5.9).

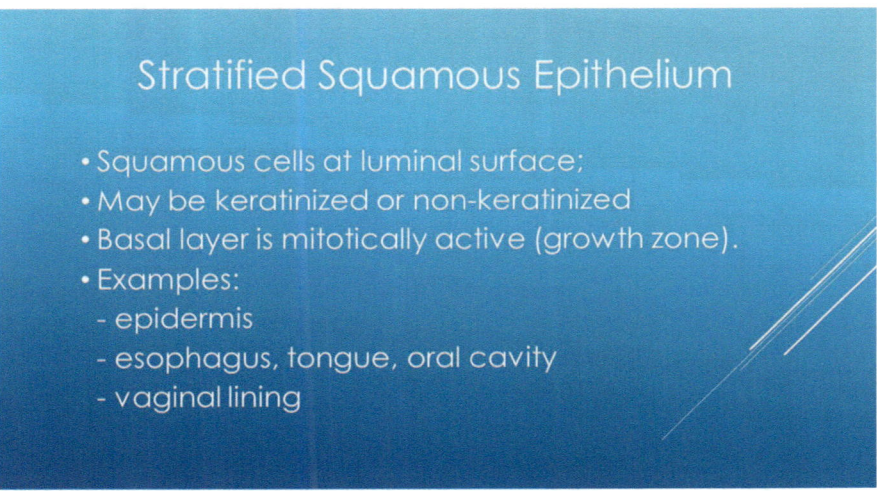

**Example 5.6**  Traditional bulleted list

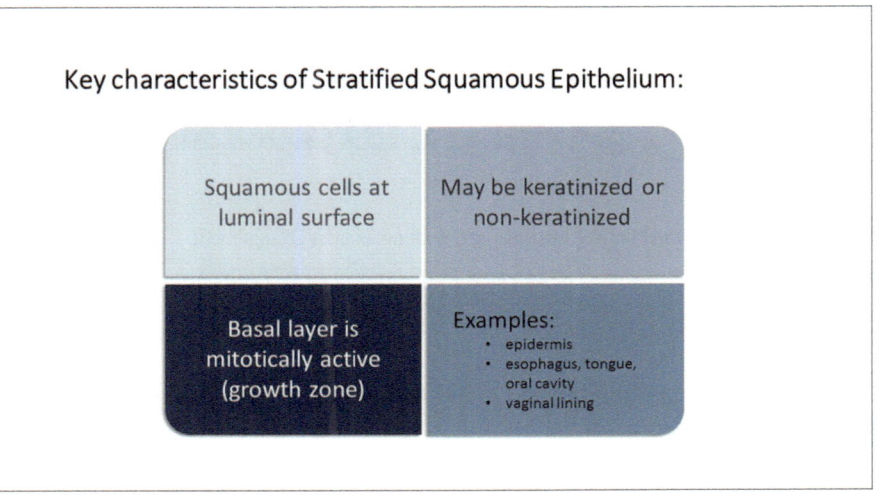

**Example 5.7**  Traditional bulleted list, revised using connected shapes

*The traditional bulleted list in Example 5.6 has been revised in Example 5.7 to emphasize the relationship between content elements. The use of connected shapes illustrates the extent to which the "list" of features together creates a cohesive whole (a type of epithelium tissue).*

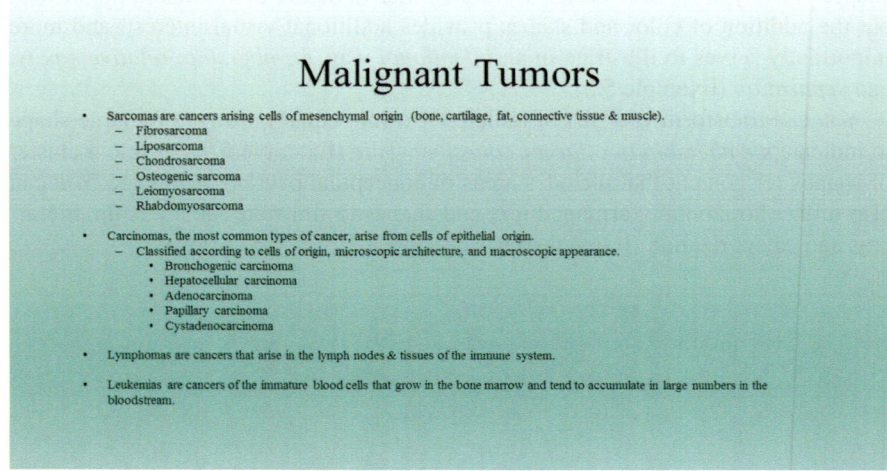

**Example 5.8**  Traditional bulleted list

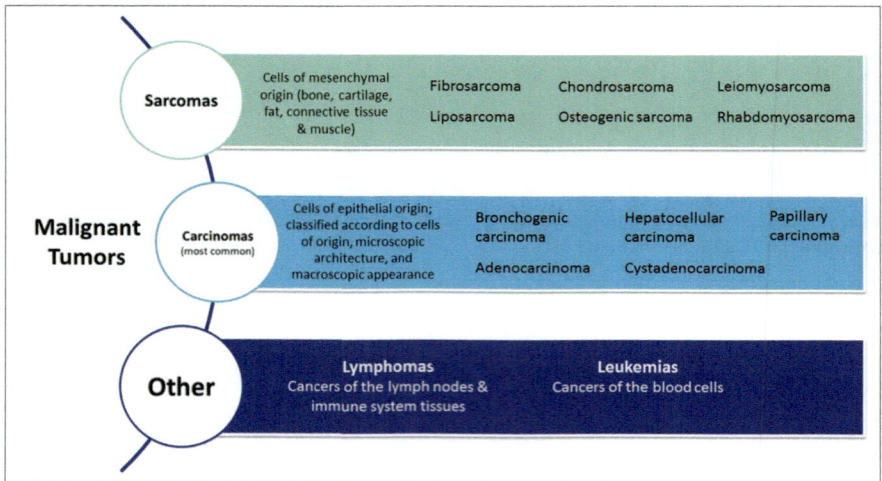

**Example 5.9**  Traditional bulleted list, revised with horizontal arrangement

*The traditional list in Example 5.8, which relies exclusively on vertically arranged text, has been revised in Example 5.9 to visually illustrate related categories of information using a primarily horizontal array of color and shapes.*

If one component of a bulleted list is actually more *important* than the others, you can use the color, size, and position of a shape to indicate this visually. The more important element will be larger in size, highlighted, or positioned in front of other, less important shapes or images (Example 5.10). Elements that are *conceptually larger*, or *greater in scope*, can be visually illustrated as such. Similarly, if one element is conceptually more *central*, position it spatially on your slide to reflect its centrality (Example 5.11).

Communicating *cause and effect, motivation, impact,* and *connection* is often more effective when done visually than with text only (Examples 5.13 and 5.15) [1, 14].

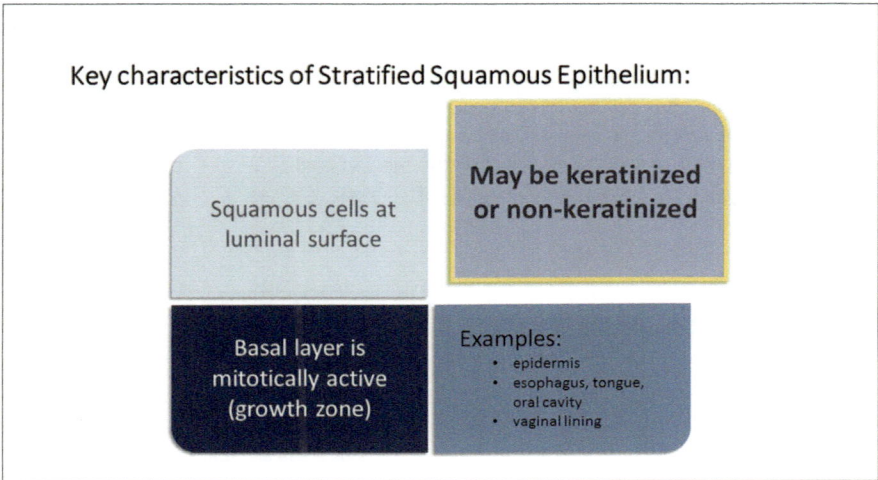

**Example 5.10** Related elements with important element emphasized

*Example 5.10 shows how you can visually illustrate the importance of one element relative to the others listed, or to highlight the element about which you are speaking at the moment.*

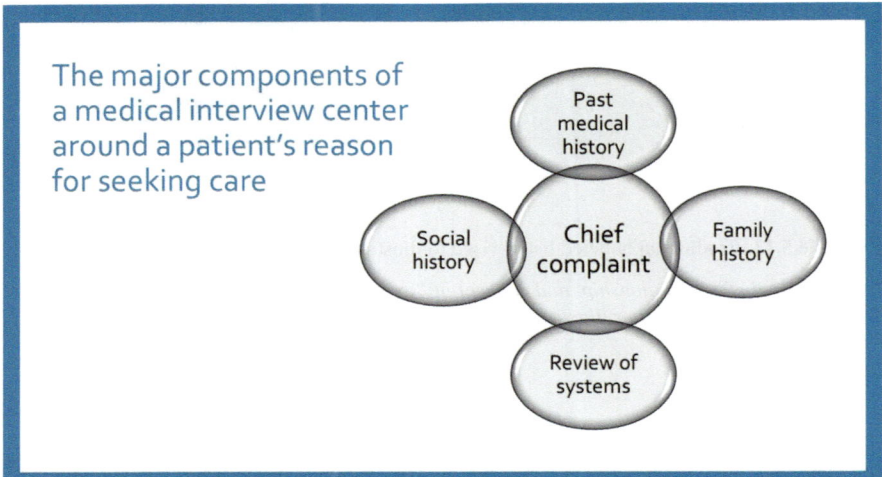

**Example 5.11** Related components around a central element

*Example 5.11 visually illustrates the centrality of the chief complaint relative to the other aspects of a patient's history.*

## Changes in Medical Education

- Motivating forces for recent change have included:
  - Societal/political movements
  - Learner advocacy
  - Issues of patient equity
  - Data re health disparities
- Resulting changes have included:
  - Increased content around health systems science
  - Increased content around social determinants of health
- Changes have been made across UME, GME & CME

**Example 5.12**  Traditional bulleted list

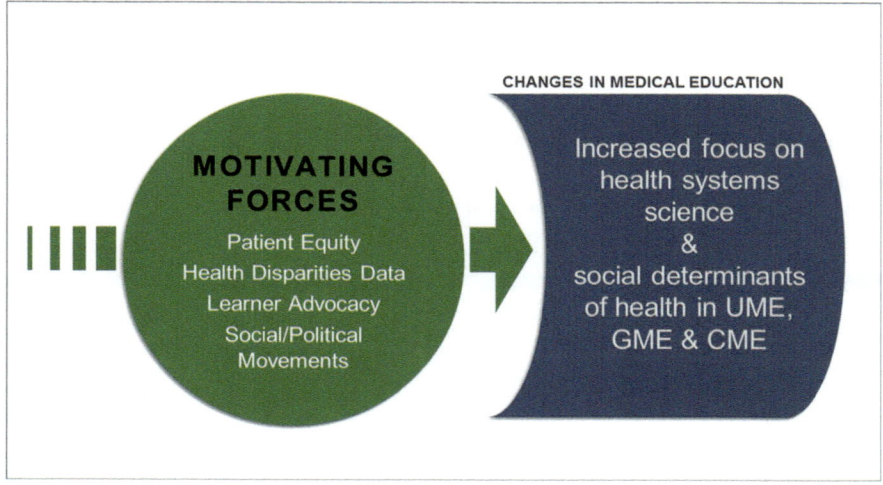

**Example 5.13**  Traditional bulleted list, revised to illustrate change and impact

*The cause and effect relationship, and concept of "impact" that is presented as a bulleted list in Example 5.12 would be better illustrated visually as in Example 5.13.*

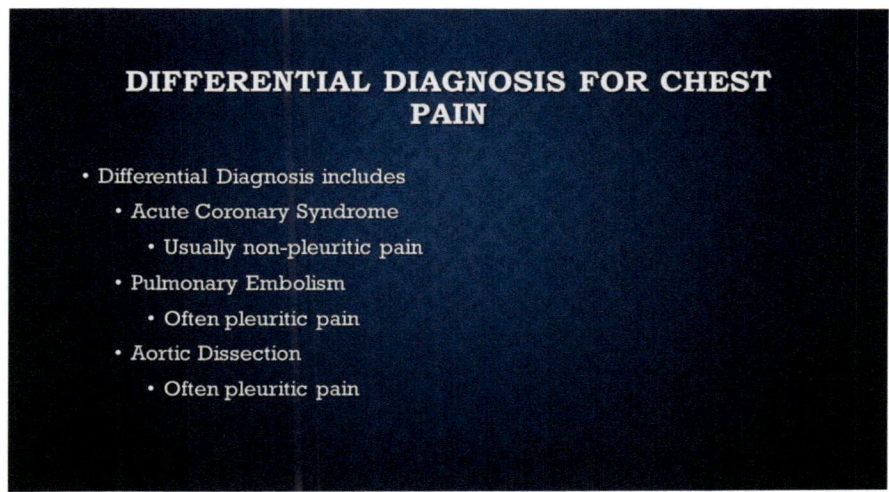

**Example 5.14** Traditional bulleted list

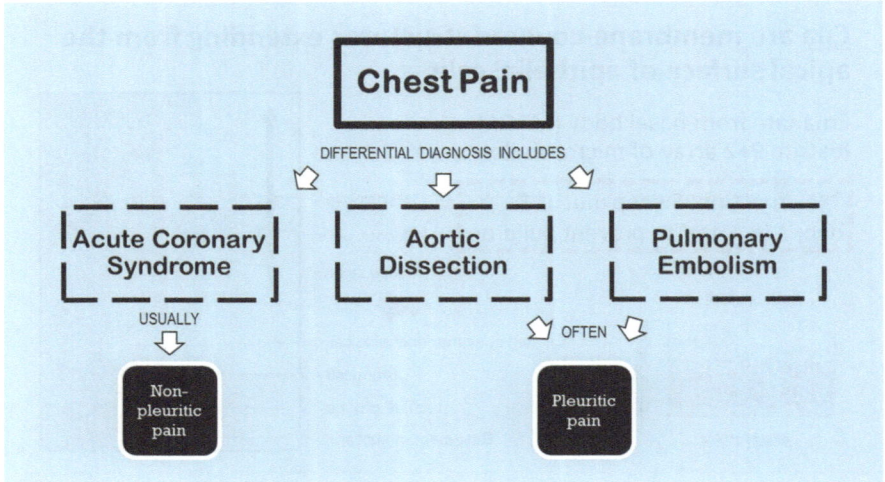

**Example 5.15** Traditional bulleted list, revised to illustrate relationships

*The thought pattern presented as a traditional linear list in Example 5.14 would be better illustrated as a "mind map" or series of connected ideas as in Example 5.15.*

When you want to call your learners' attention to one of the items on a bulleted list in order to *emphasize a point*, *expand on a concept*, or *transition to a new concept*, you can do so visually, using highlights, arrows, circles, or other visual cues (Example 5.17; see also Example 3.4 for use of arrows and shapes to highlight portions of a session outline) [7, 11].

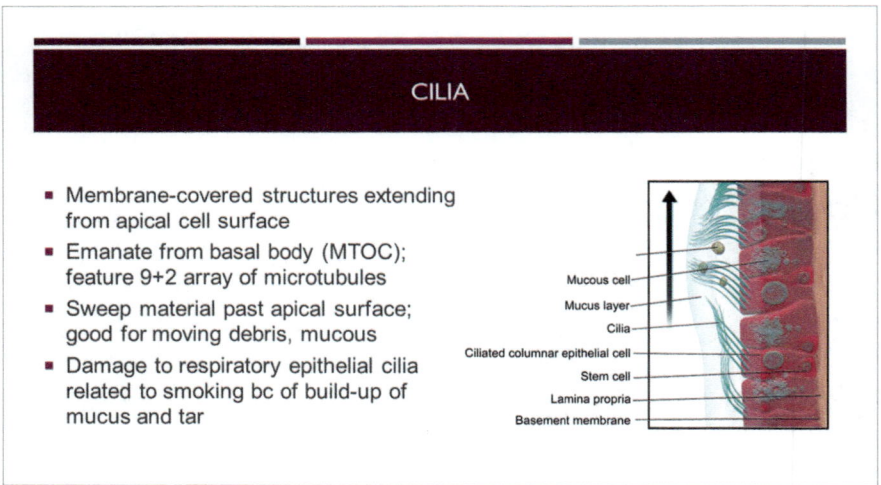

**Example 5.16**   Traditional bulleted list and image

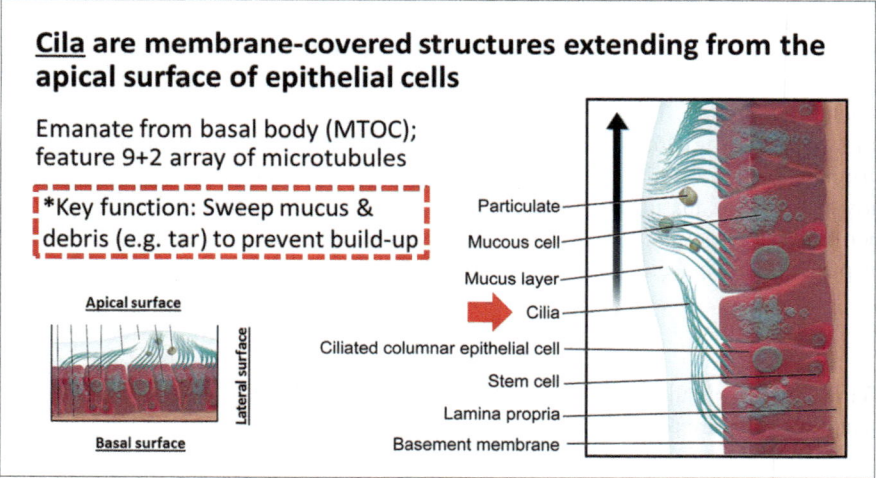

**Example 5.17**   Traditional slide design revised using assertion-evidence approach

*The traditional slide design of Example 5.16 has been revised in Example 5.17 to emphasize important content, and to visually illustrate specific spatial elements that may have been confusing to learners. Notice that the slide is still quite "busy," but the space previously allocated to an iso-lated, vague heading is now used to communicate actual information. The visual image is better utilized, and the presenter's key point is highlighted. To reduce visual overload, the presenter could easily have elements appear in a staggered fashion rather than all at once.*

You can also consider using icons or color coding to represent repeated elements within a presentation to help your learners *compare information* across slides (Examples 5.18 and 5.19). For example, if you are discussing a series of diseases, or a series of clinical findings, vital signs, or lab results for a set of cases, consider presenting that content with consistent, repeated visual cues.

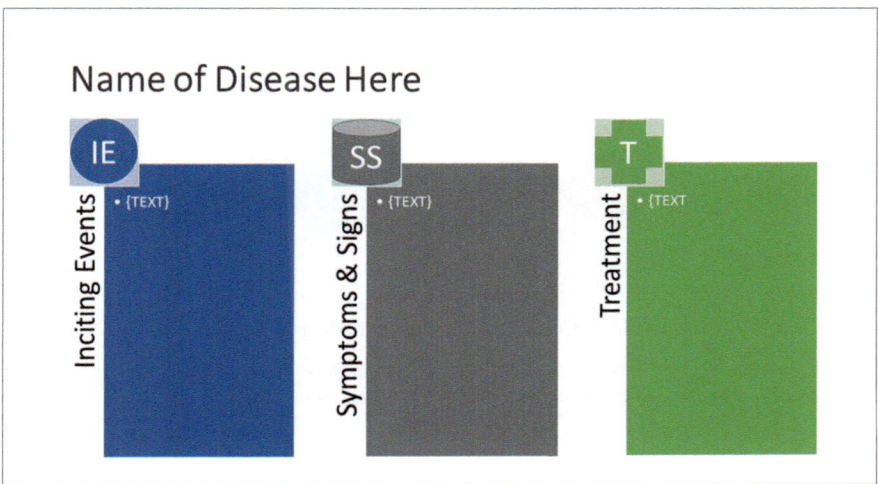

**Example 5.18**   Template slide – Comparison of diseases across slides

*Within a biomedical presentation, there are often repeated elements for different diseases, clinical cases, or sets of data. Consider creating a visual template for repeated elements (such as inciting events, symptoms, and treatment) as in Example 5.18, to facilitate easy comparison of information across slides by learners.*

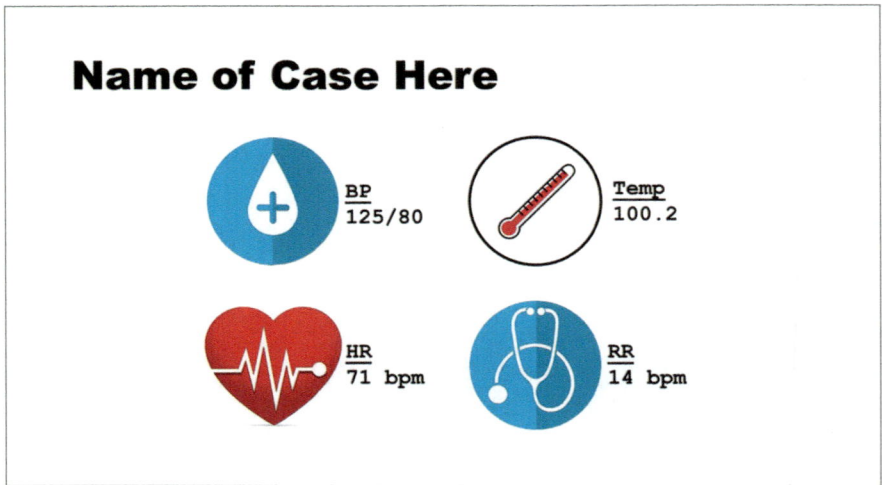

**Example 5.19**   Template slide – Comparison of clinical findings across slides

*Similar to the template in Example 5.18, Example 5.19 facilitates easy comparison of similar types of data (clinical findings) across slides via the use of visual cues and logos.*

I recently reviewed a presentation that contained summaries of a series of published studies, a common element in many biomedical presentations. The presenter wished to retain the dense bulleted text that described each study. Unfortunately after one or two of these summaries, the studies simply ran together and their relevance to his main message was difficult to discern. My advice to him was to highlight the key take-aways or conclusions from each study (see the Evidence-Assertion approach mentioned previously), and to do so using a consistent, repeated visual element (e.g., an asterisk, star, or icon) or to guide learner attention and assist in content retention.

**Timelines and Process**   If the information you include in a presentation includes a timeline or process, consider illustrating these visually (Example 5.21) [1, 11]. Passage of time and process chronology lend themselves very well to visual depiction.

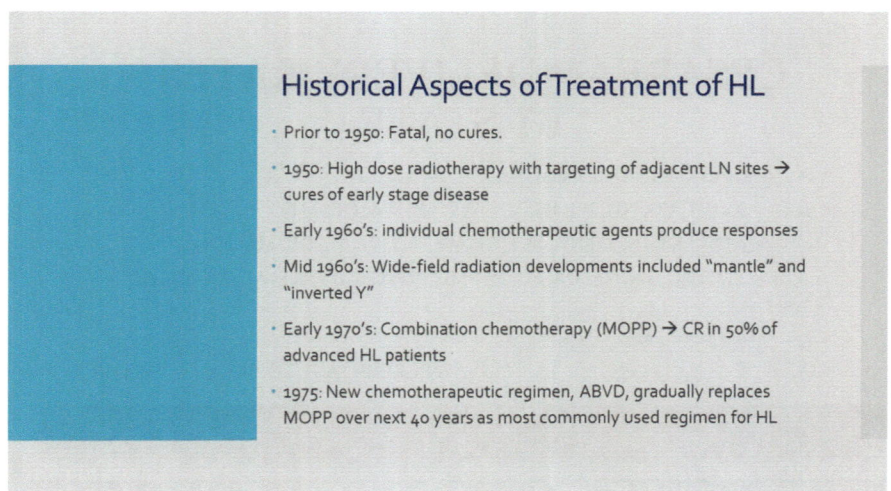

**Example 5.20**  Traditional bulleted list – Chronology

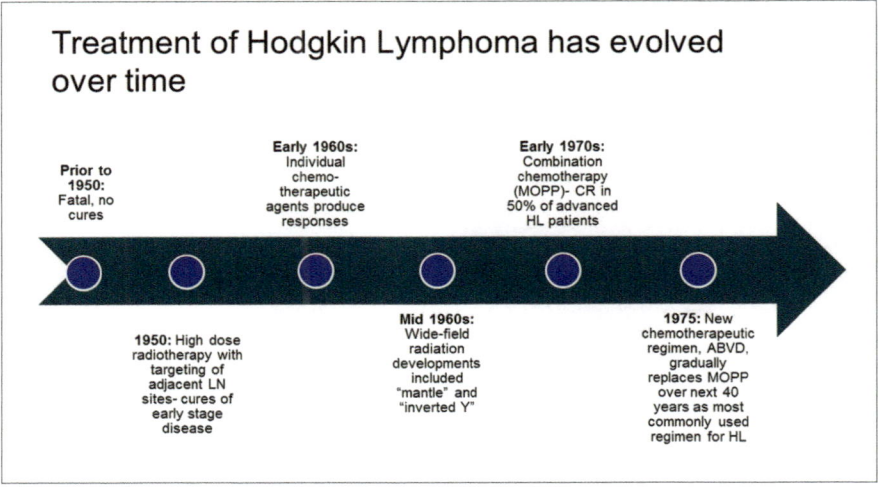

**Example 5.21**  Traditional bulleted list – Chronology, revised using timeline

*The chronology presented as a vertically arranged bulleted list in Example 5.20 is better illustrated using a horizontally arranged visual timeline like the one depicted in Example 5.21.*

**Geographical Concepts**  If your content includes geographic concepts (e.g., disease prevalence by region), consider presenting this information visually using maps (Example 5.23).

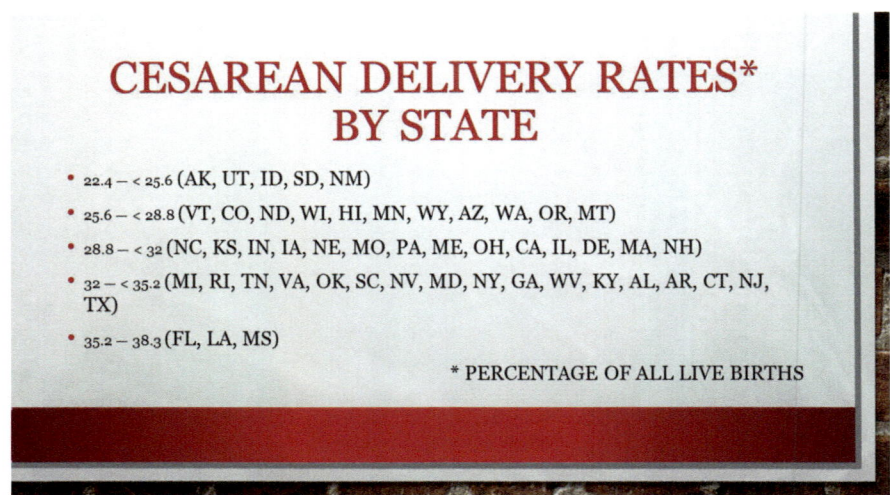

**Example 5.22**   Traditional bulleted list- Geography

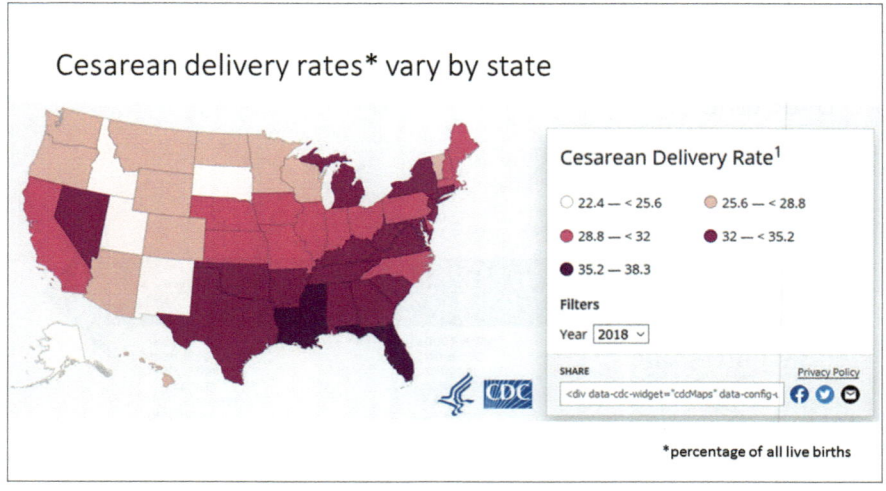

**Example 5.23**   Traditional bulleted list- Geography, revised using map

*The geographic data presented as a bulleted list in Example 5.22 is better illustrated visually using a map, as in Example 5.23 from the Centers for Disease Control.*

**Visual mnemonics**   If in your verbal presentation you use a metaphor or other mnemonic as a way to describe content, or to help learners envision a physical structure for instance, consider illustrating that metaphor visually for greatest impact.

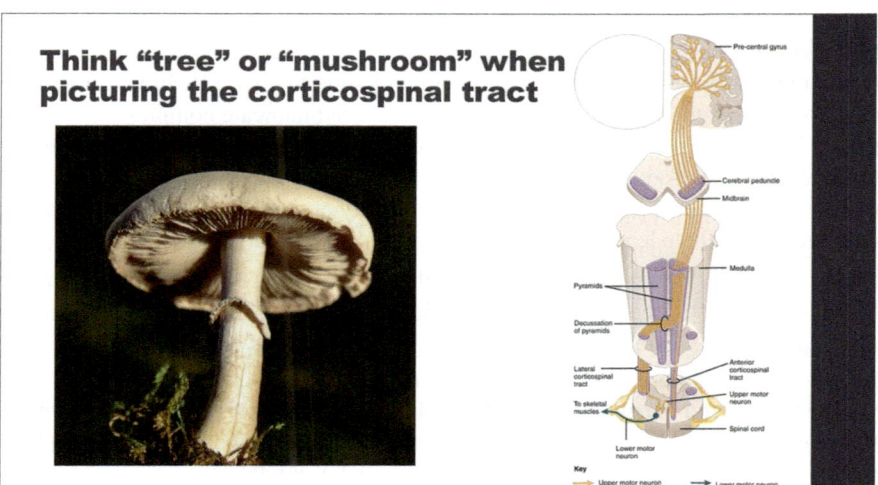

**Example 5.24**  Visual mnemonics

*Metaphors are commonly used mnemonic devices to help students visualize and retain key information. Whenever possible, illustrate these visually for maximum impact and information retention as in Example 5.24.*

The end result of reducing the amount of text on slides may be an increased number of total slides. However, limitations on slide numbers are generally arbitrary, and reflect a concern about pacing, not actual numbers. For example, Pecha Kucha, a form of community presentations that originated in Japan, uses a 20 slide limit [3, 11]. More importantly, however, each slide is visible for only 20 seconds, resulting in succinct and fast-paced communication. The number of slides does not ultimately determine presentation length-the pace of the speaker's delivery does. An increased number of slides may not result in a longer delivery, and as we will discuss in Chap. 7, any issues with timing or pacing can get worked out with appropriate delivery practice.

Medical and scientific presentations require text. Our goal is to identify appropriate opportunities to reduce, not eliminate, text, and to present information in ways that more effectively and efficiently support learner comprehension and retention.

Rule #2: *Simple is better*

Many discussions of slide design include the idea that simple is better [1–3, 5, 7, 11]. For the most part, I agree. Simple *is* better when it comes to background templates, font types, and color schemes. I mention each of these design elements below. However, I do want to differentiate the kind of simplification used as part of business or marketing, from the kind that is useful in education.

Much of business-based communication is about identifying a unified and singular message. The business world has created various "rules" about the number of words that can appear on a slide, or on a line of slide text [2, 11]. In education, we need to develop good communication in order to communicate complexity, not simplicity. We cannot, and should not, try to adhere to arbitrary quantitative "rules" about slide design. Therefore, while I advocate for simple slide design, I do so in order to make visual and conceptual room for the complexity of our content, and of the knowledge we want to help learners construct. "A concise presentation allows the learner to build a coherent mental representation – that is, to focus on the key elements and to mentally organize them in a way that makes sense" (Mayer, 2009, p. 106).

**Templates**   There are many slide design templates out there that are fun and colorful, and include interesting fonts. However, be aware that the more "interesting" your template, and the more "extras" you add to it, the more distracted a learner may be from your actual content. As you can see from the revised examples I include in this book, I prefer plain, usually light colored, backgrounds.

**Fonts**   Generally speaking, you should choose a "sans serif" font, such as Calibri or Arial, rather than a serif font, such as Times New Roman or Georgia. Letters in serif fonts have extra little lines or "feet" that make them harder to read, especially from far away. I recommend that you stay away from script-based and italicized fonts for the same reason.

---

- Arial is a sans-serif font, and is a good choice

- Calibri is another sans-serif font, and is also a good choice

- Serif fonts, like Times New Roman, can be more difficult to read, especially from a distance

- Other things that make text more difficult to read include:
  - FONTS IN ALL CAPS
  - *Italicized fonts*
  - *Script-based fonts*

- "Informal" fonts such as Comic Sans may not be appropriate for all academic presentations

---

**Example 5.25**   Font styles

*As you can see in Example 5.25, some fonts involve more stylistic flourishes and are thus potentially more difficult to read, especially from a distance or when projection quality is poor. They can therefore add an unnecessary cognitive burden on your learners.*

**Contrasting Colors** You should also choose a high contrast color scheme. Very light font on a very dark background works well, but is hard on printers if your plan is to distribute copies of your slides. I tend to prefer a very dark font on a very light background, which has the added advantage of being easily annotated in either paper or iPad version.

**Example 5.26** Poor color scheme 1

**Example 5.27** Poor color scheme 2

*The color schemes in Examples 5.26 and 5.27 make content difficult to read, and therefore act as a distraction, add to learners' cognitive load, and ultimately impede learning.*

Rule #3: *Visual elements should be relevant and informative*

One unfortunate consequence of asking presenters to decrease their reliance on text-based slide design is a subsequent increase in the use of decorative template designs, "funny" clip-art images, or random word art. I tend to discourage the use of clip-art and other stylistic flourishes on the grounds that they are usually not relevant to the content, and are potentially distracting. When images are extraneous to the core concepts being presented, they may engage learners' precious cognitive energy in unintended ways, and distract learners from important content [7, 15, 16]. "The coherence design [of multimedia learning] is to avoid seemingly interesting words, pictures, and sounds that are not relevant to the lesson's main message" (Mayer, 2009, p. 106).

Clip-art, and images cut and pasted from the results of an online search, can also be inadvertently inappropriate in nature. I frequently see "pirated" images in academic presentations without appropriate attribution, and images that are too casual for a serious presentation (Example 5.28).

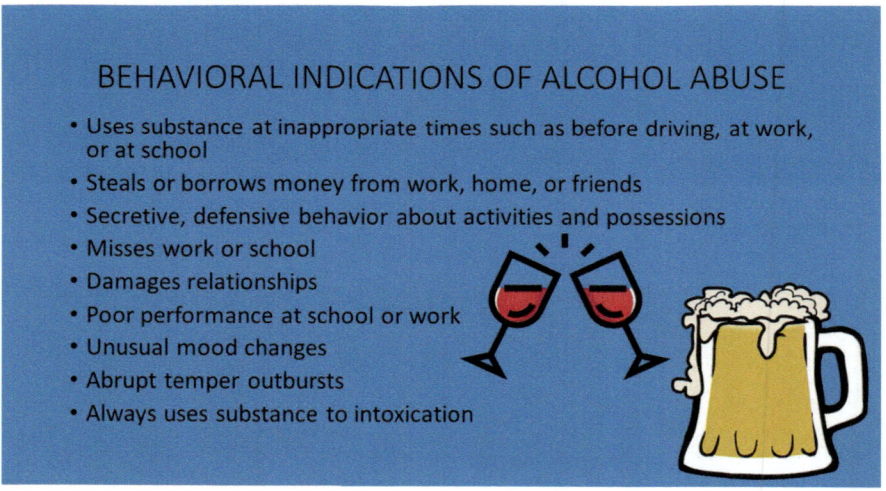

**Example 5.28**  Inappropriate clip-art

*In this Example of a traditional bulleted list, the presenter tried to create "visual interest" using generic clip-art. However, the clip-art images do not serve any educational or illustrative purpose, and are inappropriate given the seriousness of the slide content.*

Generally speaking, images should only be included on a slide if they are relevant to the content at hand, and/or provide supportive information [1, 5, 7]. Anything else is a distraction. Institutional logos should be included on a title slide, but are not necessary (and are potentially distracting) on subsequent slides [2, 11]. Likewise, slide numbers are generally not useful (with the exception I mention in Chap. 3) and should be eliminated.

Rule #4: *Text and visual elements should be large and readable*

All text and visual elements such as diagrams, graphs, or tables (as well as their labels and keys), should be large enough to be read and understood from the back of a large room [1, 3, 5]. All visual aids should be of good quality, and not fuzzy or hard to read (Example 5.29). When in doubt, make your images as big as they can get without negatively impacting their quality.

Moreover, visual elements may need to be manipulated to emphasize, or even exaggerate, important content in order to promote knowledge acquisition and retention [15, 16]. "Faithful" visual representations may not actually be the most efficient learning tools. For example, for novice learners, actual human cadavers may need to be supplemented by high-quality print or electronic anatomical representations in order to help learners identify basic structures. You could consider tracing the outline of certain structures to emphasize shape or location (Example 5.30), increasing the contrast or changing the color of an image using editing tools in order to direct

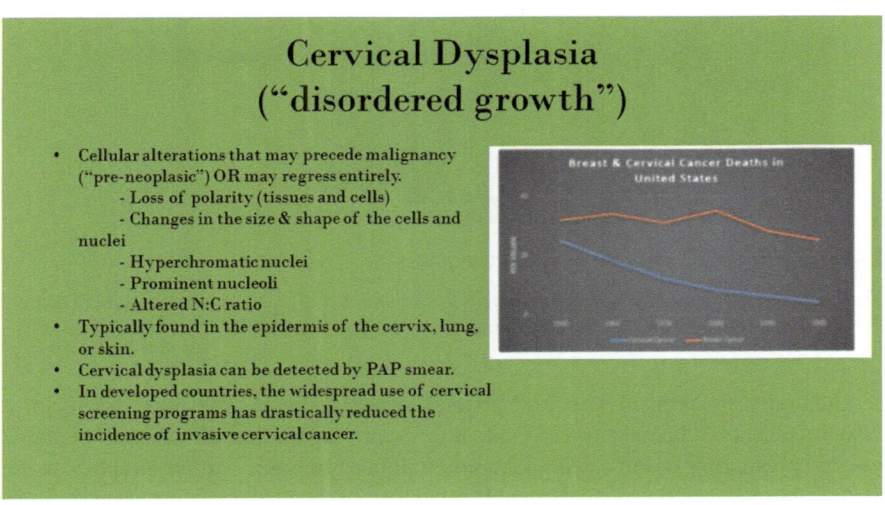

**Example 5.29**  Poor quality visual image

*In addition to an unattractive color scheme and serif font, this slide suffers from a poor-quality image that is out of focus and too small, which makes it difficult to read and ultimately educationally useless.*

learner attention, or as mentioned previously, insert shapes or arrows to highlight important visual elements (Examples 3.3, 5.17).

By packaging information effectively, and by visually emphasizing the most salient information, you can "reduce the cognitive load without reducing the amount of information conveyed to the learner" (Dror, 2011, p. 292).

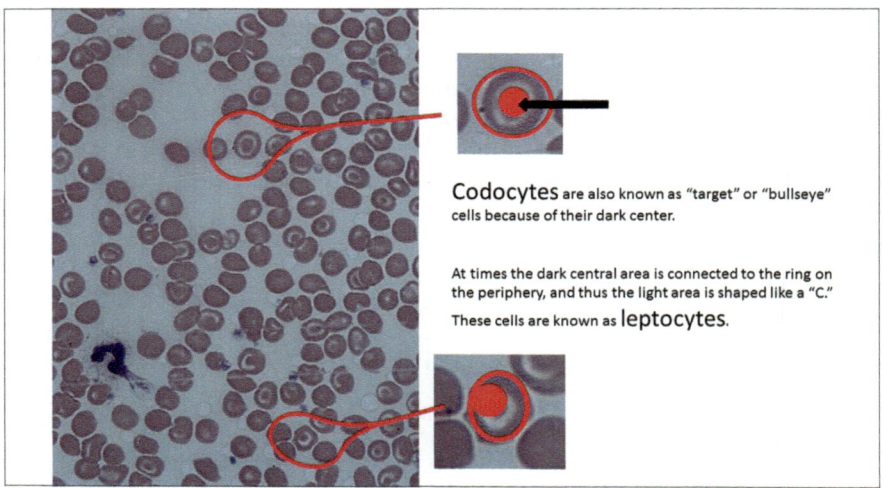

**Example 5.30**   Visual emphasis of salient information

*The use of color, shapes, and magnified images in Example 5.30 serve to emphasize salient content for learners to promote knowledge acquisition and retention.*

Generally speaking if you find yourself apologizing for the poor quality of a visual, you should take the time to redo it *prior* to your next presentation. If the table you are presenting is dense with data, you will need to guide learner attention using arrows, circles, or other visual cues. If much of the data in a table or graph is actually irrelevant, consider creating an excerpt of the table from scratch, and use that to present the relevant data to learners (with appropriate attribution of course).

Similarly, if you have clipped and pasted an excerpt from a written text, but the image is blurry, you should consider retyping the excerpt directly into your slide. (If you dread retyping the text, take that feeling of dread as a sign that the text is too long and should be edited down!)

Rule #5: *Your slides should include color, space, and a variety of images*

A very talented presenter, Dr. Angela Anderson, gave the best, and simplest, piece of advice I have ever heard about slide design. She advised faculty to view their PowerPoint presentations on "slide sorter" ("grid view" in Google Slides) as a way of checking for overall use of color, space, and visual interest [2, 5, 11]. If your slides are too text-heavy, you will see a sea of black and white. Now practice the "instructional empathy" I mentioned in Chap. 3 and imagine being on the receiving end of those endless black-and-white slides. Imagine how difficult it would be to pay attention when every slide looks exactly like the previous one.

By making simple changes to some of our text-based slides, we create whole presentations that are visually more varied and engaging. We also combat some of the shortcomings of presentation software default designs by enhancing and reducing text, and visually communicating important abstract concepts that are often missing from traditional text-based slides. In these ways, we transform our conventional presentations into *healthy presentations*.

**Summary Points**
- The anatomy of a presentation includes your verbal delivery (what you say), your visual delivery (what you show), and supplemental materials (what you provide).
- Use supplemental materials to facilitate asynchronous learning and to reduce the amount of text included in your visual delivery.
- Use text (especially in the slide heading) to help your learners understand the main "assertion" you are making about the content at hand.
- Bulleted lists fail to indicate the relative importance of information listed, the relationship between the pieces of information, and the relationship of those pieces to the slide heading.
- Use shapes, color, and diagrams to visually illustrate, and better communicate, the complex information that is traditionally included in bulleted lists.
- Use visual images and diagrams to better illustrate information regarding time-lines, processes, stages, geographic information, and visual metaphors.
- When it comes to slide design and templates, simple is better.
- Remove any visual elements that are not directly relevant or informative.
- Enlarge or recreate visual elements (such as tables or diagrams) so that they are easily read by your audience.
- Check your presentation for the use of color, space, and images.

# References

1. Nathans-Kelly T, Nicometo CG. Slide rules: design, build, and archive presentations in the engineering and technical fields, vol. 3. Hoboken: Wiley; 2014.
2. Atkinson C. Beyond bullet points: using Microsoft PowerPoint to create presentations that inform, motivate, and inspire (Bpg-other). Microsoft Press; 2005.
3. Alley M. The craft of scientific presentations: critical steps to succeed and critical errors to avoid. 2nd ed. New York: Springer; 2013.
4. Kernbach S, Bresciani S. 10 years after Tufte's "Cognitive Style of PowerPoint": synthesizing its constraining qualities. In: 2013 17th international conference on information visualisation. IEEE; 2013, July. p. 345–50.

5. Reynolds G. Presentation Zen design: a simple visual approach to presenting in today's world. Berkeley: Pearson Education; 2014.
6. Tufte ER. The cognitive style of PowerPoint. New York: AP/Wide World Photos; 2003.
7. Mayer RE. Multimedia learning. Cambridge: Cambridge University Press; 2009.
8. Garner JK, Alley MP, Sawarynski LE, Wolfe KL, Zappe SE. Assertion-evidence slides appear to lead to better comprehension and recall of more complex concepts. In: ASEE annual conference and exposition, conference proceedings; 2011.
9. Garner J, Alley M. How the design of presentation slides affects audience comprehension: a case for the assertion-evidence approach. Int J Eng Educ. 2013;29(6):1564–79.
10. Morrison M. How to create a better research poster in less time. 2019. https://www.youtube.com/watch?v=1RwJbhkCA58. Accessed 9.23.20.
11. Duarte N. Slide: ology: the art and science of creating great presentations, vol. 1. Sebastapol: O'Reilly Media; 2008.
12. Barr RB, Tagg J. From teaching to learning—a new paradigm for undergraduate education. Change: The Magazine of Higher Learning. 1995;27(6):12–26.
13. Wiggins GP, McTighe J. Understanding by Design. Alexandria: Association for Supervision and Curriculum Development; 1998.
14. Lang JM. Small teaching: everyday lessons from the science of learning. San Francisco: Wiley; 2016.
15. Dror I, Schmidt P, O'connor L. A cognitive perspective on technology enhanced learning in medical training: great opportunities, pitfalls and challenges. Med Teach. 2011;33(4):291–6.
16. Dror IE, Stevenage SV, Ashworth AR. Helping the cognitive system learn: exaggerating distinctiveness and uniqueness. Appl Cogn Psychol. 2008;22(4):573–84.

# Chapter 6
# Reviewing Slides for Diversity and Inclusion

**Abstract**
This chapter recognizes and endorses efforts in medical and health professions education to promote diversity and inclusive teaching practices. It encourages educators to review their teaching and teaching materials for a diversity of images, and for use of inclusive language. This chapter explicates the intersection of good slide design, and the ways in which we talk about racial categories when it comes to disease risk and prevalence. *Healthy presentations* communicate an updated understanding of race as a social construct, and require that presenters talk explicitly about the racial categories they cite, the origin of those racial categories, and their clinical relevance.

Recently, medical schools have begun to pay an unprecedented, and long overdue, amount of attention to the way we teach about race and medicine. On a macro-level, medical education institutions are engaging in large-scale reviews of their curricula in order to ensure that new generations of clinicians have the most accurate and precise information available to them, and that the patient care they ultimately provide is as equitable and bias-free as possible [1–6]. On a micro-level, individual faculty are engaging in reviews of their presentations for issues of diversity and inclusion along a variety of dimensions such as age, ability, sex, gender, and ethnicity.

Inclusive teaching practices, ones that create a welcoming learning environment and that reflect the biomedical and social experiences of individuals across groups and cultures, involve all three aspects of our presentations – our verbal and visual deliveries, and the information we include in our supplementary materials. (See Chap. 5 for more about the anatomy of a presentation). Even the most well-meaning faculty may require practical guidance as to changes they can make to their teaching and teaching materials to be more inclusive, and to reflect an anti-racist orientation.

E. P. Green, *Healthy Presentations*, https://doi.org/10.1007/978-3-030-72756-7_6

## 6.1 Diversity of Images

The most straightforward way to increase the inclusivity of your presentations is to use a diversity of images that depict individuals of varied gender, age, and skin color. These images may not always be easy to find, and you may need to access specialized publications [7, 8].

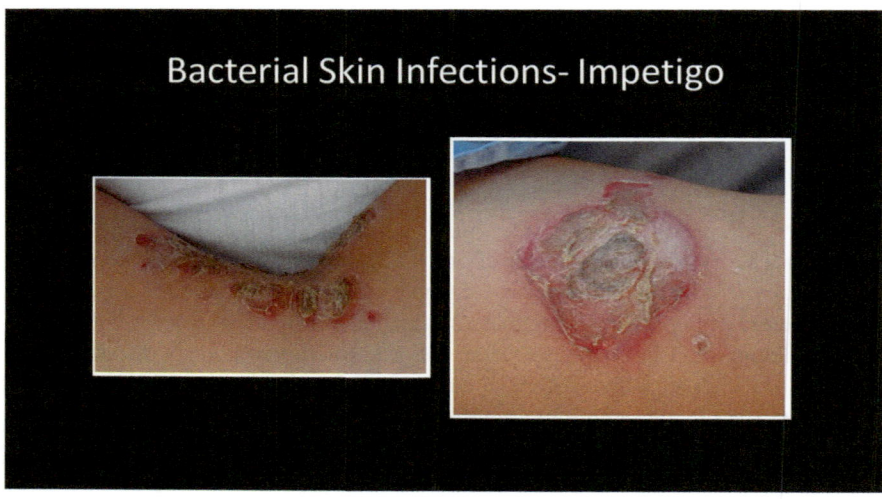

**Example 6.1** Homogeneous images. (Page 179 Dermatology Atlas for Skin of Color. Figures 31.4 and 31.5)

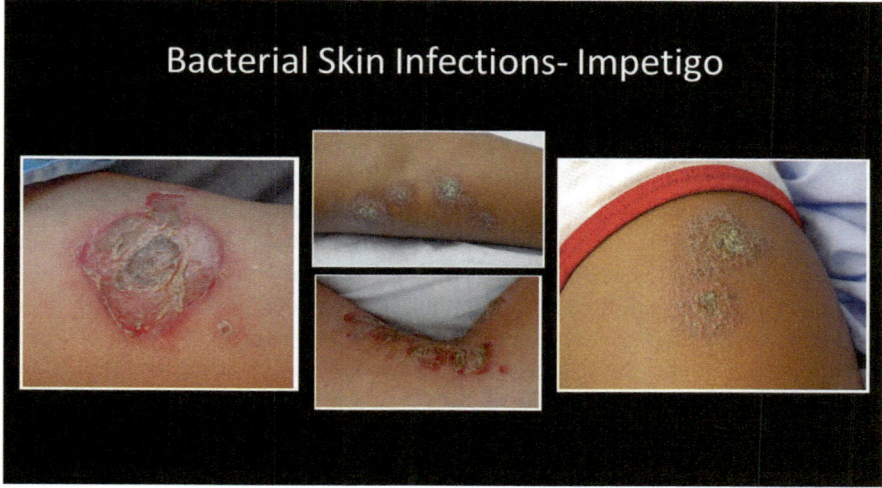

**Example 6.2** Heterogeneous images. (Page 179 Dermatology Atlas for Skin of Color. Figures 31.1, 31.2, 31.4 and 31.5)

*The slide shown in Example 6.1 was revised to be more inclusive of a range of skin tones in Example 6.2.*

The images you include as examples of "typical" pathology should be diverse enough so as to prevent stereotyping [2]. This may be especially important for pathology associated with some level of social stigma. For example, only including images of young people when discussing STIs may give the impression that only young people are at risk. If only young people are thought to be at risk, older individuals may then miss out on essential screenings.

The use of diverse images may seem inconsequential in terms of the actual facilitation of learning, but in reality it can have an enormous impact on learning and learners. The use of diverse images can help novice clinicians think broadly about diagnoses in actual patients. It can help prevent diagnostic "shortcuts" [9–11] in which clinicians prematurely rule out potential diagnoses based on limited or biased assumptions about the patient's race, ethnicity, age, or gender. Diverse images can also help your diverse audience feel engaged in the learning process when they see images that reflect themselves, their families, and their communities. The ability to create personal connections with content, and to see the relevance of information to one's own life, is a central tenet of adult learning [12, 13].

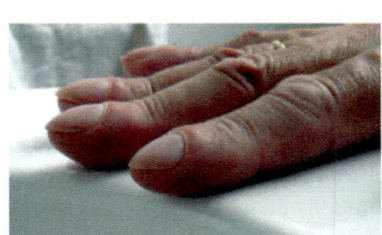
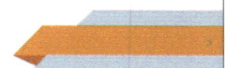
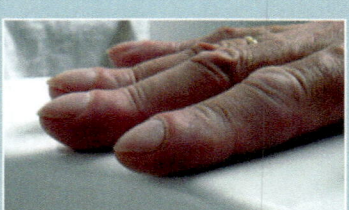

**Example 6.3**   Single "representative" image

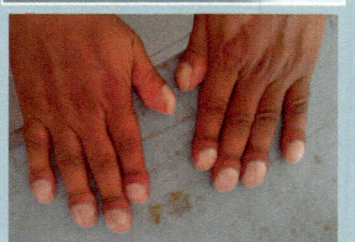

**Example 6.4**   Increased diversity of images

*The slide shown in Example 6.3 was revised to be more inclusive in Example 6.4. Not only was an additional image added, the presenter also altered a description of how a patient's skin may appear, to make it more inclusive of a range of skin tones.*

When we think about the images we use, we should also consider the clip-art and graphics we include. As mentioned in Chap. 5, I discourage the use of clip-art on the grounds that it is usually not relevant to the content, and tends to be distracting [14–16]. However, there are times when use of a stock photo or clip-art image is illustrious, or appropriately humorous, and we should be intentional about the diversity of those images across a presentation as well.

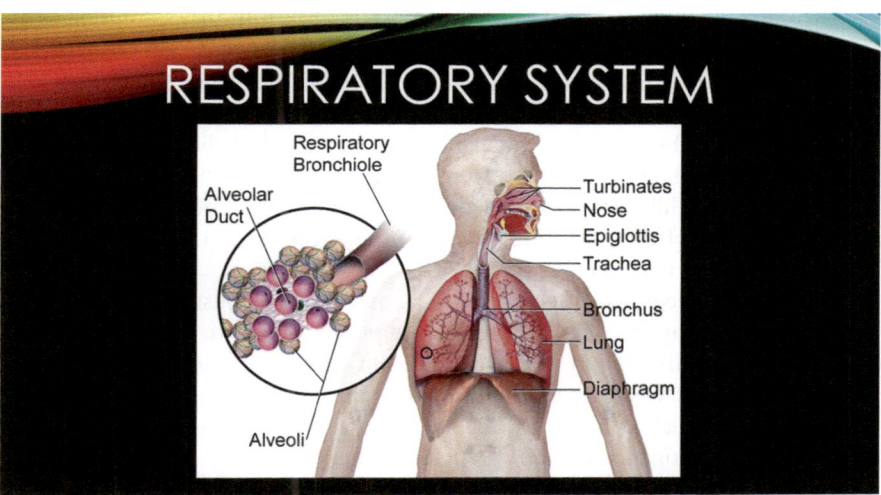

**Example 6.5**   Diversity in clip-art

*The slide depicted in Example 6.5 would be improved by a more subtle background design, and potentially by an image that depicts an individual from a minority population particularly if other images within the presentation uniformly depict male gender and/or white skin.*

## 6.2   Inclusivity of Language and Terminology

A review of our presentations for inclusivity and bias should also attend to the language and terminology we use, in both our verbal delivery and in our presentation materials, including slide text. As we know, the words we use (and do not use) have great power, and our roles as educators require us to use them thoughtfully and with care [17, 18].

> **Key Point**
> Inclusive teaching practices involve being very intentional about the language we include in, and omit from, our presentations.

For example, use of inclusive language in medical education acknowledges that individuals in the audience may also be patients themselves [19, 20]. Exclusively using "they" to refer to patients, and "we" to refer to providers can exacerbate the patient-provider divide, especially when talking about something like mental illness or surviving trauma. Our learners, and their loved ones, have all potentially experienced the medical system in the role of patient at some point in time.

I once observed a compassionate lecturer of medical students describe with great sensitivity the difference between population-level and individual-level statistics when it comes to cancer survival rates. She did so purposefully, in recognition of the number of young people in the audience who were likely to have parents or grandparents diagnosed with some form of cancer. I also observed a presenter talk to that same group, using dire language, about the impact of herpes infections on newborns. No discernable attention was paid to the statistical likelihood that many of the 20–30-year-olds in his audience were infected with the virus, or that over half were women of childbearing age. A sensitivity to these issues might prevent learners from "turning off" or "shutting down" during a lecture, and thus would have a significant positive impact on learning.

Clinical language is also often value-laden, out-of-date, or just imprecise in ways that we do not always recognize, especially in presentations we have given repeatedly, but have not thoroughly reviewed in recent years. For example, we may use imprecise language when we equate different populations, comparing populations from a *continent*, such as Africa or Asia, with populations from a much smaller, and possibly more homogeneous *country*, such as Poland.

**Substitute updated terminology to be more inclusive - Abbreviated list**
Substitute "differences" for "irregularities"
Substitute "typical" for "normal" (excluding laboratory values)
Substitute "intellectual disability" for "mental retardation"
Substitute "transgender" for "transexual"

Inclusive and antiracist teaching calls for a reexamination of the way in which we talk about race and medicine more generally. Discussions in the medical education literature indicate an increasing understanding of racial categories as social, rather than biological, constructs [1, 4–6, 21]. Different countries use very different census categories and terminology to reflect relevant "race" and ethnicity. The very nature of racial categories, and government-sponsored racial identification, changes as we move across borders, and continues to change *within* national boundaries over time [22–26]. In light of evolving and inconsistent definitions and understanding of racial categories, we need to thoroughly review the data we provide to learners.

## 6.3  Review of Citations

Another potential area for review is your reference list, to make sure that the official guidelines and research you cite are up to date. In order to provide learners with complete and accurate information, you should be able explain the way in which particular studies account for race, and the limitations of those methodologies [2]. Many time when race is mentioned, it is actually being used as a substitute for something else. Common social conceptions of race are conflated with other identifying elements such as ethnicity (shared culture and language), country of origin, or skin color.

Before we present data to our learners, we should look at them critically to ensure that we understand and can explain what exactly they do and do not reflect. We should ask ourselves a series of questions about the very content in which we consider ourselves to have expertise.

**Questions for consideration**
- Do the studies you cite account for individuals who identify as biracial or as "two or more races" (as they do in the US census)?
- Can you explain if the studies you cite define race by self-report, census data, medical record review, or some other method, and the implications of each?
- Are there differences between the official clinical guidelines and recommendations that you cite, and how you actually practice? (If there are, this may be an opportunity to use these differences as a point of discussion with your learners to encourage unbiased clinical practice).
- Can you explain why race, and not socioeconomic factors, is the relevant influence in a particular study? For example, when discussing a study about the incidence of diabetes in certain populations, are you able to describe the role of genetics versus socioeconomic factors?

As scientists, physicians, and educators we should strive to be as specific, accurate, and bias-free as possible. When the answers to these questions are unclear or unaccounted for, we must say so.

A rethinking of how we conceptualize race requires a reconsideration of how we incorporate racial categories into medical education as a part of case studies, presentations of data regarding risk for particular diseases, and as we train learners to craft clinical presentations [3–5, 27, 28]. Continuing to perpetuate the notion of race as a biological construct may increase learner bias and perpetuate flawed clinical practices [4, 5, 27, 28].

## 6.4    Race as a Risk Factor

Traditional presentations of race in biomedical presentations highlight the shortcomings of presentation software default settings [29, 30]. Racial categories tend to be included on undifferentiated bulleted lists of risk factors for disease, but "membership" on that list is the only meaning a learner can infer. Any nuance to these sentence fragments is lost, as are the potential relationships between them. Additional information, such as more specific classification of different factors, information about which risks are more clinically salient, or how risk is actually determined, is needed.

There exist real points of alignment between the improvements we can make to our slide design as detailed in Chap. 5, and improvements we can make to our teaching practices and materials to make them more inclusive. As we redesign our slides to escape the constraints of traditional templates, we can also make changes to the ways in which we present racial categories as related to risk and prevalence.

**Key Point**
When racial categories appear on an undifferentiated bulleted list, learners are unable to adequately or appropriately infer meaning and/or relevance.

Often race, in and of itself, is not a risk factor for disease – it is acting as a surrogate for a combination of socioeconomic factors including racism, income, and access to care, as well as behaviors, some of which are culturally based, including diet [31–33]. You can see that multiple factors are listed on the slide in Example 6.7, but behavioral and demographic information are all jumbled together in a way that leads to learner confusion. In this instance, a bulleted list slide design is particularly ineffective in conveying the complex contributions to risk of stroke.

## STROKE
## RISK FACTORS

- Hypertension
- Diabetes Mellitus
- Smoking
- Obesity
- Prior stroke
- Family history
- Hyperlipidemia
- Carotid Stenosis
- Low birth weight

- Physical inactivity
- African American
- Hispanic
- Alcohol use
- Asian
- Diet

**Example 6.6**   Race as a risk factor– Traditional bulleted list

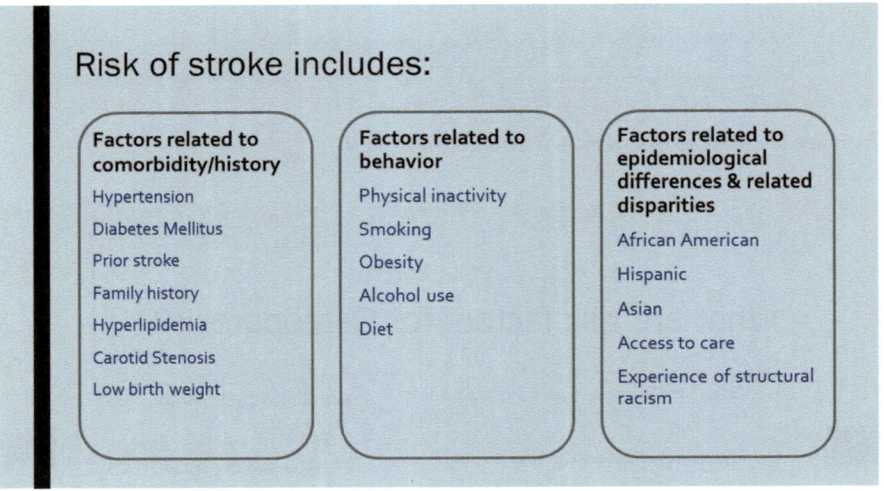

**Example 6.7**   Race as a risk factor – Traditional bulleted list, revised

*In Example 6.6, several common (very broad) racial categories are listed as risk factors for stroke within a classic undifferentiated bulleted list. This represents a very common understanding of stroke by clinicians. The revised slide in Example 6.7 includes a more accurate and detailed description of factors that contribute to risk of stroke.*

When we talk about disease being more prevalent in one population versus another, or if we talk about racial categories as risk factors for certain diseases, we need to be specific about *why*. Minor changes to the slide on stroke in Example 6.7, separating out behavioral factors from ones that are epidemiological in nature or related to comorbidity, make the information presented more specific and more accurate. These changes do not necessarily address the core issue of race as a social versus biological construct, but a presenter could easily mention in her verbal delivery the fact that she includes these terms to represent self-identification in common socially accepted categories, *not* as an endorsement of a biological basis for race.

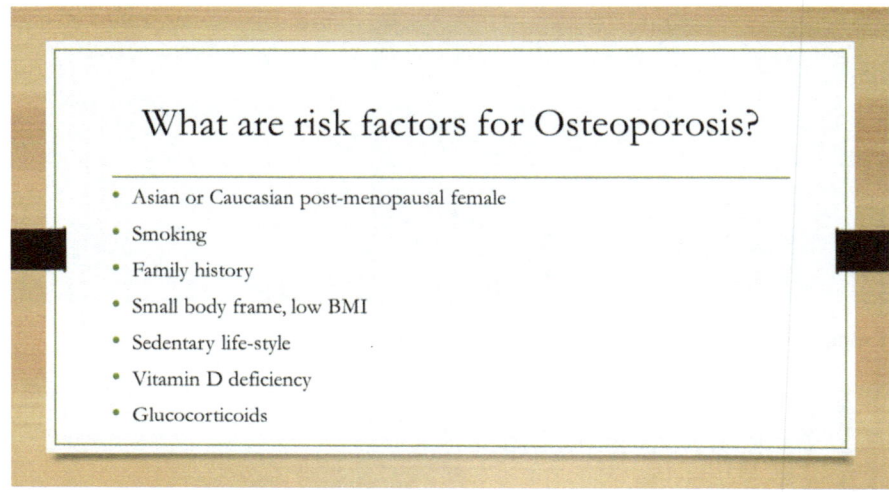

**Example 6.8**   Race as risk factor – Traditional bulleted list

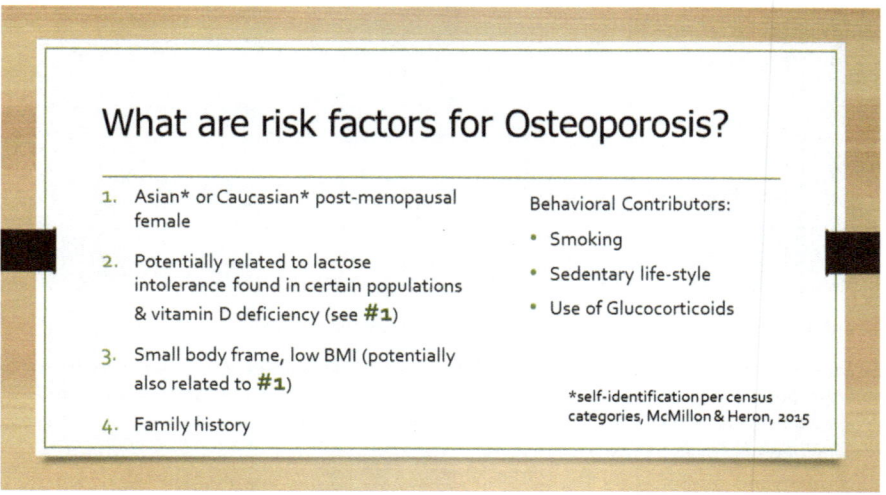

**Example 6.9**   Race as risk factor – Traditional bulleted list, revised

*The slide presented in Example 6.8 was revised to (1) differentiate between behavioral and other categories of risk, (2) more clearly indicate the relationship between some of the factors listed which were unclear on the original undifferentiated bulleted list, and (3) include additional information about the origin of the racial categories listed.*

It may be that when we present information using race, we are simply reporting the results of a study that categorized participants using socially accepted terminology. But again, our job is to be as specific and as accurate as possible. If your slide cites categories utilized in a study where patients self-identified as being part of a particular racial group, you should say exactly that (Example 6.9).

## 6.5   Prevalence by Racial Category

You may also want to review your presentations for information about disease prevalence broken down by racial categories. Disease prevalence across racial groups is a common slide in biomedical presentations, and the data displayed can be very useful to highlight health disparities or, as I mentioned above, when one population is at greater potential risk than another. However if the data are presented via an undifferentiated bulleted list without clarifying details, a learner might assume that certain racial groups are just biologically or genetically more likely to experience a particular disease than others. This is generally not the case, in part because common racial categories are not biological in nature, and thus do not necessarily indicate genetic commonalities. Simple changes to verbal and visual delivery can clarify what prevalence statistics actually reflect.

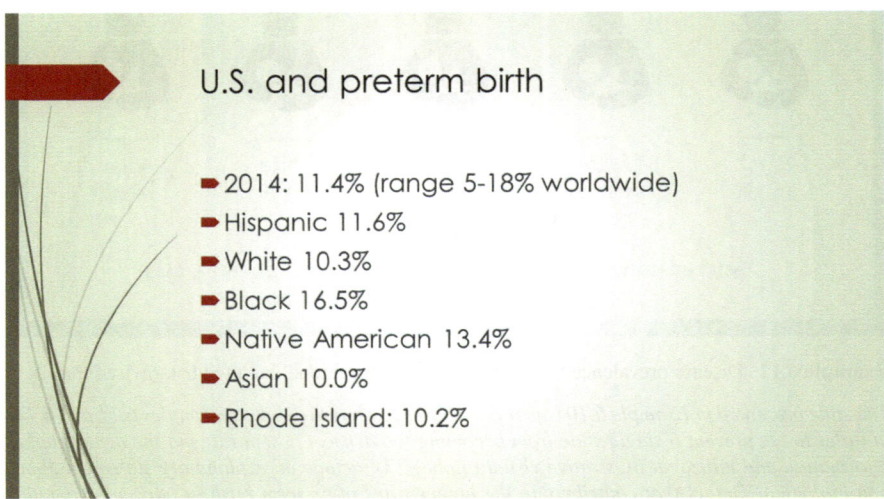

**Example 6.10**  Disease prevalence by racial category – Traditional bulleted list

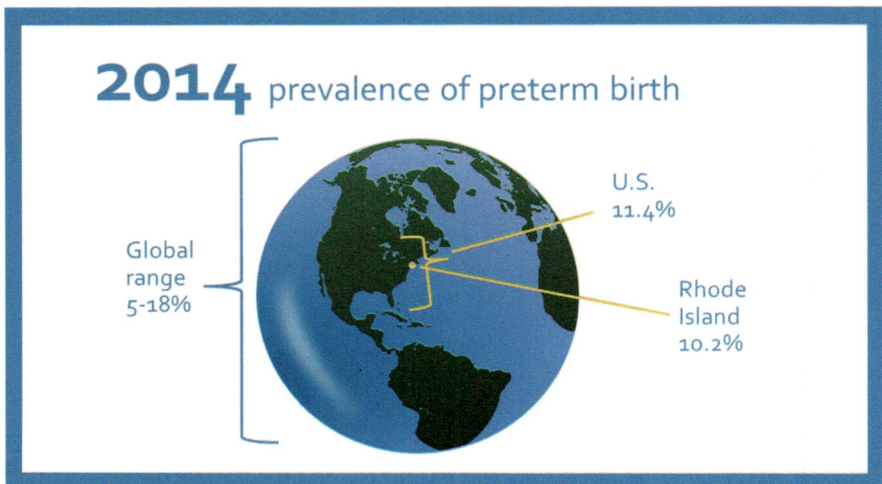

**Example 6.11**   Disease prevalence by racial category – Traditional bulleted list, revised Part 1

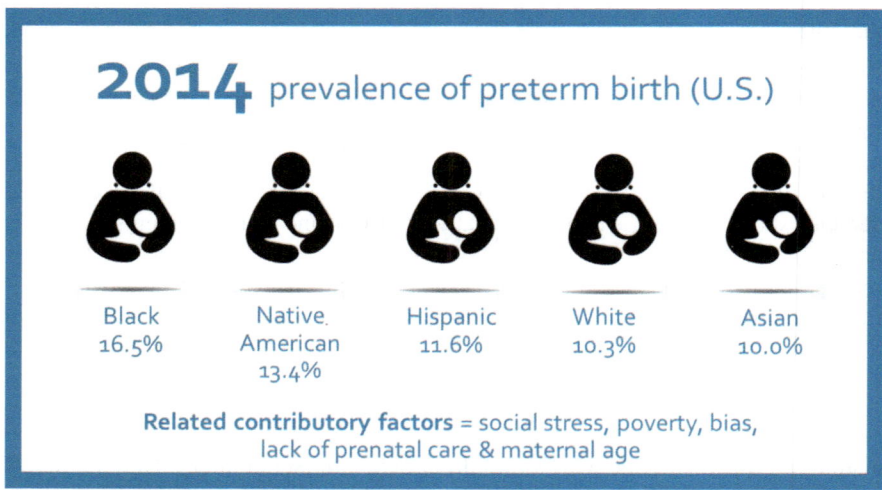

**Example 6.12**   Disease prevalence by racial category – Traditional bulleted list, revised Part 2

*The slide presented in Example 6.10 was revised into two separate slides (Examples 6.11 and 6.12) in order to (1) prevent a single slide from becoming too dense, (2) separate out the demographic information and utilize an illustrative visual (globe), (3) include an explanatory statement about non-biological factors that contribute to the higher rates of preterm birth in particular popula-tions, and (4) decrease reliance on a bulleted list.*

If indeed you are referencing shared geographic ancestry and genetic markers, as is the case for sickle cell disease (which occurs in individuals with ancestors from equatorial areas including Africa, Turkey, Greece, India, Asia, Saudi Arabia, Latin America, and the Caribbean), consider incorporating a map into your slide to illustrate geographic origins as was done in Examples 5.23 and 6.11. Reducing genetically based disease prevalence to racial categories on an bulleted list could lead novice clinicians to inappropriately limit their genetic screenings and diagnoses based on a misguided and overly simplistic conception of "race."

## 6.6   Range of Possible Edits

There are a range of possible edits you can make to your materials and to your verbal delivery when considering inclusivity. The suggestions provided in this chapter are not meant to restrict faculty in terms of what they can present, or the words they can use. The suggestions are certainly not meant to detract from faculty expertise. I include them here as potential tools to improve instruction, and therefore improve learning.

**Explain (or Eliminate)**  The simplest option is to take out information about race and identity if it is irrelevant to the issue at hand. It is worth asking yourself if the information you present about the race, gender expression, gender identity, or sexual orientation of a patient is actually important. Are the descriptive terms you use informative clinically? Do they impact your treatment plan or management of care? If the answer to these questions is "no," consider removing the information from your presentation.

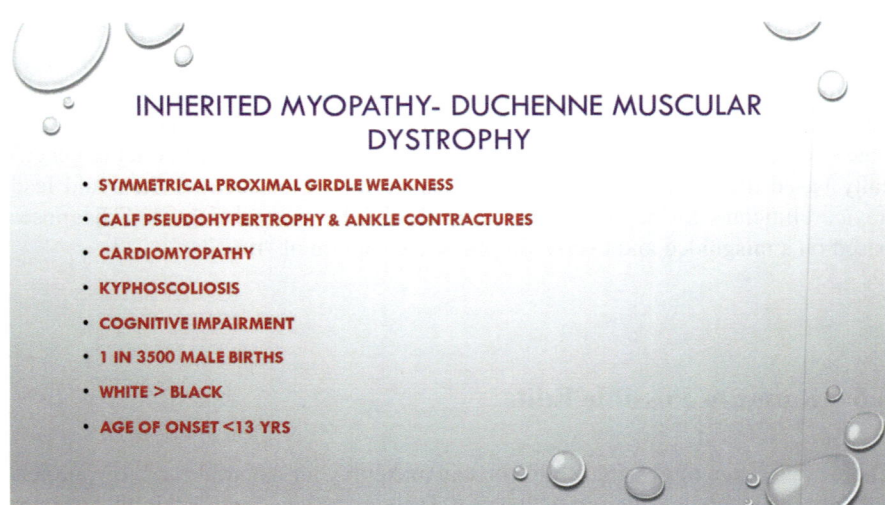

INHERITED MYOPATHY- DUCHENNE MUSCULAR
DYSTROPHY

- SYMMETRICAL PROXIMAL GIRDLE WEAKNESS
- CALF PSEUDOHYPERTROPHY & ANKLE CONTRACTURES
- CARDIOMYOPATHY
- KYPHOSCOLIOSIS
- COGNITIVE IMPAIRMENT
- 1 IN 3500 MALE BIRTHS
- WHITE > BLACK
- AGE OF ONSET <13 YRS

**Example 6.13**  Race as irrelevant information

*In this Example, the relative prevalence of Duchenne muscular dystrophy in white patients versus black patients is indicated, but without specific numbers, or definitions of the broad racial categories mentioned. No explanation is provided about factors that contribute to a difference in prevalence, or how this information might change treatment. Learners are potentially left with questions regarding whether white patients are simply receiving more medical care for the condition. In this case, removing any mention of race would be a reasonable edit to make (along with improving the font color and slide background!).*

It is certainly not the goal of this chapter to encourage faculty to avoid talking about race altogether. The overarching message is that *if you include racially based information, be prepared to talk explicitly with learners about where it comes from, what it means, and why it is important.*

**Consider a "Disclosure"**  Another possible approach to creating inclusive presentations is to provide information to your learners ahead of time about the data you are presenting. In Example 6.14, the presenter wanted to make sure that his audience understood his thoughtful approach to sex and gender, and he framed that part of his presentation as a "disclosure" about the origins of his data.

## Disclosure regarding terminology & data used

During this lecture on sexually transmitted infections (STIs), I will primarily be drawing from medical literature, and using language, that has historically focused on cisgender persons and cisgender anatomy. This is in no way meant to discount transgender persons. You can extrapolate certain risks for STIs to various populations based on current anatomy, contact, and sexual behaviors.

For those interested in other populations, the CDC publishes its STI guidelines every 4 years, which has included gender and sexual minority populations.

The medical literature also continues to grow with increasing attention to STIs in gender and sexual minority communities.

**Example 6.14**  Disclosure

*By including this "disclosure" at the beginning of his presentation, the presenter (1) reassured the audience that he was not unaware of issues related to the treatment of transgender patients, (2) appropriately indicated that his data and terminology come from traditional sources that may not reflect minority populations, and (3) provided suggestions of sources for more up-to-date information.*

**Define Your Terms**  You could also frame additional information as a "definition of terms" to help your learners understand exactly what you mean, and how and why you are using particular words or phrases. In Example 6.15, the presenter wanted her learners to know what she meant by certain labels, and she alerted her learners that she would try to help them understand the relevance of this information throughout her talk.

## Definition of terms used

• The term "intellectual disability" refers specifically to standard IQ test results in the range of 50-70 (mild) and 35-50 (moderate).

• The term "developmental delay" refers to a delay in meeting specific behavioral milestones aligned with chronological age.

• The term "advanced maternal age" refers to mothers over the age of 35 at the time of pregnancy.

Whenever possible I will try to clarify the origins of terminology used, and we will discuss clinical implications of this information.

**Example 6.15** Definition of terms

*By including this initial slide, the presenter (1) provided specific definitions of the terms used in subsequent slides, and (2) reassured her audience that efforts would be made during her presentation to clarify their clinical importance whenever possible.*

Given our understanding of the shortcomings inherent in traditional presentations of complex information [15, 29, 30, 34], and given our increasing awareness of the ways in which medicine and medical education perpetuate systemic racism and exclusionary practices of all kinds [1, 3–5, 27, 35], it is important for faculty to review their teaching practices and materials through a new and critical lens. A review of our presentations for diversity of images, inclusive language, and explicit critique of our data and sources, is a wonderful place to start.

The way we traditionally present information about race and identity is a perfect example of why we need to make changes to our slide design (see Chap. 5). Learners need more and better information than bulleted lists can provide. *Healthy presentations* communicate an updated understanding of race as a social construct, and help learners to construct knowledge that is accurate and inclusive.

**Summary Points**
- Review your teaching materials and practices for inclusive images and language.
- Review the studies and data you cite so that you can clearly communicate to your learners how relevant racial categories are defined, and any rationale for their inclusion.
- Avoid undifferentiated bulleted lists that include racial categories when presenting risk factors for disease or disease prevalence.
- If you include racially based information in your presentation, be prepared to talk explicitly with learners about its origin, meaning, and clinical relevance.

# References

1. Anderson MR, Moscou S, Fulchon C, Neuspiel DR. The role of race in the clinical presentation. Fam Med-Kansas City. 2001;33(6):430–4.
2. Guidelines for Promoting a Bias-Free Curriculum [Internet]. Vagelos College of Physicians and Surgeons. Vagelos College of Physicians and Surgeons; 2018 [cited 2019Oct28]. Available from: https://www.ps.columbia.edu/education/student-resources/honor-code-and-policies/guidelines-promoting-bias-free-curriculum.
3. Krishnan A, Rabinowitz M, Ziminsky A, Scott SM, Chretien KC. Addressing race, culture, and structural inequality in medical education: a guide for revising teaching cases. Acad Med. 2019;94(4):550–5.
4. Tsai J, Ucik L, Baldwin N, Hasslinger C, George P. Race matters? Examining and rethinking race portrayal in preclinical medical education. Acad Med. 2016;91(7):916–20.
5. Tsai J, Crawford-Roberts A. A call for critical race theory in medical education. Acad Med. 2017;92(8):1072–3.
6. Yudell M, Roberts D, DeSalle R, Tishkoff S. Taking race out of human genetics. Science. 2016;351(6273):564–5.
7. Jackson-Richards D, Pandya AG, editors. Dermatology atlas for skin of color. Berlin, Heidelberg: Springer; 2014.
8. Taylor SSC, Serrano AMA, Kelly AP, Lim H. Taylor and Kelly's dermatology for skin of color. New York: McGraw-Hill; 2016.
9. Braun LT, Zwaan L, Kiesewetter J, Fischer MR, Schmidmaier R. Diagnostic errors by medical students: results of a prospective qualitative study. BMC Med Educ. 2017;17(1):191.
10. Graber ML, Franklin N, Gordon R. Diagnostic error in internal medicine. Arch Intern Med. 2005;165(13):1493–9.
11. Krupat E, Wormwood J, Schwartzstein RM, Richards JB. Avoiding premature closure and reaching diagnostic accuracy: some key predictive factors. Med Educ. 2017;51(11):1127–37.
12. Knowles MS. Self-directed learning: a guide for learners and teachers. Chicago: Association Press; 1975.
13. Merriam SB, Caffarella R, Baumgartner S. Learning in adulthood: A comprehensive guide. 3rd ed. San Francisco: Jossey-Bass; 2007.
14. Mayer RE. Multimedia learning. Cambridge: Cambridge University Press; 2009.
15. Nathans-Kelly T, Nicometo CG. Slide rules: design, build, and archive presentations in the engineering and technical fields, vol. 3. Hoboken: Wiley; 2014.
16. Reynolds G. Presentation Zen design: a simple visual approach to presenting in today's world. Berkeley: Pearson Education; 2014.
17. Goddu AP, O'Conor KJ, Lanzkron S, Saheed MO, Saha S, Peek ME, et al. Do words matter? Stigmatizing language and the transmission of bias in the medical record. J Gen Intern Med. 2018;33(5):685–91.
18. Matson CC, Beck LA, Rajasekaran SK. Using language that reflects who is the center of our care. Acad Med. 2019;94(9):1400.
19. McKevitt C, Morgan M. Illness doesn't belong to us. J R Soc Med. 1997;90(9):491–5.
20. Woolf K, Cave J, McManus IC, Dacre JE. It gives you an understanding you can't get from any book.'The relationship between medical students' and doctors' personal illness experiences and their performance: a qualitative and quantitative study. BMC Med Educ. 2007;7(1):50.
21. Hoffman KM, Trawalter S, Axt JR, Oliver MN. Racial bias in pain assessment and treatment recommendations, and false beliefs about biological differences between blacks and whites. Proc Natl Acad Sci. 2016;113(16):4296–301.
22. Bennett C. Racial categories used in the decennial censuses, 1790 to the present. Gov Inf Q. 2000;17(2):161–80.
23. Brown A. The changing categories the US has used to measure race. Pew Research Center. 2015;7(3):15.
24. Carvalho JAMD, Wood CH, Andrade FCD. Estimating the stability of census-based racial/ethnic classifications: the case of Brazil. Popul Stud. 2004;58(3):331–43.

25. King-O'Riain RC. Counting on theCeltic Tiger' adding ethnic census categories in the Republic of Ireland. Ethnicities. 2007;7(4):516–42.
26. Sandefur GD, Campbell ME, Eggerling-Boeck J. Racial and ethnic identification, official classifications, and health disparities. Critical perspectives on racial and ethnic differences in health in late life. 2004; 25–52.
27. Acquaviva KD, Mintz M. Perspective: are we teaching racial profiling? The dangers of subjective determinations of race and ethnicity in case presentations. Acad Med. 2010;85(4):702–5.
28. Vyas DA, Eisenstein LG, Jones DS. Hidden in plain sight—reconsidering the use of race correction in clinical algorithms. N Eng J Med. 2020;383:874.
29. Kernbach S, Bresciani S. 10 years after Tufte's" cognitive style of PowerPoint": synthesizing its constraining qualities. In: 2013 17th international conference on information visualisation. IEEE; 2013, July. p. 345–50.
30. Tufte ER. The cognitive style of PowerPoint. New York: AP/Wide World Photos; 2003.
31. Brondolo E, Love EE, Pencille M, Schoenthaler A, Ogedegbe G. Racism and hypertension: a review of the empirical evidence and implications for clinical practice. Am J Hypertens. 2011;24(5):518–29.
32. Trent M, Dooley DG, Dougé J. The impact of racism on child and adolescent health. Pediatrics. 2019;144(2):e20191765.
33. Williams DR, Lawrence JA, Davis BA. Racism and health: evidence and needed research. Annu Rev Public Health. 2019;40:105–25.
34. Alley M. The craft of scientific presentations: critical steps to succeed and critical errors to avoid. 2nd ed. New York: Springer; 2013.
35. Marte D. Can a woman of color trust medical education? Acad Med. 2019;94(7):928–30.

# Chapter 7
# The Delivery

**Abstract**
This chapter describes important steps to take before, during, and after your presentation. It makes the case that practicing out loud beforehand is key to presentation success. A *healthy presentation* is defined as one that is reviewed, revised, and saved appropriately.

In Chap. 5, I talked about the three parts of a presentation – your verbal delivery (what you say), your visual delivery (what you show), and your supplemental materials (what you provide). In order to "deliver" a good presentation both verbally and visually, there are important things to consider before, during, and after you clip on a microphone, load up your slides, and begin to speak.

## 7.1 In Preparation (Before)

**Know Your Learners** As I mentioned in Chap. 3, it is essential that you target your presentation to the learners at hand [1, 2]. The level of detail and conceptual complexity you include in your talk will be very different for an audience of first-year medical students than it will be for a group of your peers at a national conference. Similarly, what and how you teach that group of peers, all of whom are experienced, knowledgeable professionals, will differ from a teaching session with a heterogeneous group of sub-interns, residents, fellows, and physician assistant trainees. Basic information about your learners, who they are, their general level of mastery, and group size and composition, should all inform the development of learning objectives, and the choice of content and teaching strategies. (See Chap. 3

E. P. Green, *Healthy Presentations*, https://doi.org/10.1007/978-3-030-72756-7_7

for more on learning objectives, and Chap. 4 for more on teaching strategies that facilitate active learning.)

**Know the Context**  It is not always possible to identify exactly what your learners do and do not know. But many times it *is* possible to ascertain the locus of your talk within the broader educational context. Consider asking curriculum or program directors what lectures precede and follow yours, so you have a sense of where your information fits within a broader curriculum. Does the session on interpreting chest X-rays come before or after your presentation on interpreting EKGs? Inquire of a conference organizer if there are other talks related to your topic being presented as well, so you have a sense of the audience's potential experience and exposure to similar content.

Inquire ahead of time about the physical space in which you will be presenting. Many carefully planned workshop activities have been thwarted because venue seating does not allow for small groups, or the acoustics in the room do not permit participants to hear each other properly.

Logistical issues such as the availability of a slide advancer, or the ability to play videos with sound, should also be investigated prior to the time of your presentation. Unexpected complications such as poor projection quality can necessitate last minute slide changes to color schemes or font sizes. Early morning or post-lunch presentation time slots may necessitate additional activities to engage sleepy learners!

**Most Importantly, Practice**  There is an enormous chasm between the organization and clarity of the thoughts in your head, and the organization and clarity of the words that come out of your mouth. In our heads, we are articulate – our voices are confident, our descriptions and explanations are eloquent. The slides we have designed so carefully are so familiar to us now that we are lulled into a false sense of security that the words will just magically flow from our mouths to the waiting ears of our audience. Too often, this magical scenario fails to appear. In reality, we may stumble over our words. Our voices, so confident in our minds, newly shake with nervousness. Our descriptions and explanations fall short.

> **Key Point**
> "Practicing" a talk too often involves a silent review of slides. Deliver your content *out loud* at least once or twice before your actual presentation.

The only way to bridge the chasm between your thoughts and your words is to practice [1, 3]. Out loud. Repeatedly. Be the crazy lady talking to herself as she drives home. Be the crazy guy muttering to himself on a long walk. Even better, ask a trusted colleague to listen to your presentation and give you feedback. Ask if your institution's office of faculty development offers an observation service like the Talk Review and Feedback sessions I conduct with faculty.

Videotape and watch your presentation ahead of time. While potentially painful (we are often our own worst critics!), this process can be very useful. Watching yourself can be a way to identify and eliminate any verbal tics (such as "umm" or "like") that we sometimes use as "fillers" when we are unsure of word choice, or of the best way to express our ideas. Once you are aware of these tics you can be more intentional about your word choice and expression of ideas in subsequent practice sessions.

Verbalizing your thoughts, with special attention to beginnings, endings, and other content transitions, will go a long way to ensure a smooth delivery. Practice has the additional benefit of reducing public speaking anxiety as your confidence in your ability to deliver a wonderful presentation grows.

## 7.2   In the Moment (During)

Congratulations, the hard work of crafting a thoughtful presentation has already been done! Your job now is much simpler. As I mentioned in Chap. 3, you are the expert on your content. You have done your due diligence, and gotten a sense of your audience and their level of knowledge. Even if you are surrounded by experts in the field, have confidence that you know the particular arrangement and interpretation of information you are about to convey better than anyone. Your job now is to lead the audience through that information. Remember that your presentation is not about you, it is about the learning it can help facilitate. Your slides are just tools to help facilitate that learning.

**Audience Goodwill**   One key thing to keep in mind is that your audience *wants* you to succeed. They *want* to see your passion. They *want* you to lead them confidently through your materials.

Realizing the extent of an audience's goodwill was a turning point in my own development as a presenter. At a conference composed of brief back-to-back presentations, I had the opportunity to compare the emotional experience of being in the audience of a highly confident presenter, with the emotional experience of being in the audience of the next presenter who was visibly nervous. The former was invigorating, the latter was anxiety provoking and highly uncomfortable. My body became tense, and I found myself wanting to supply the presenter with the words she was so clearly seeking. I cringed at her stumbles and felt her discomfort. Yet I celebrated her occasional clear explanation, and genuinely applauded at the visible relief with which she ended her presentation. *If only as a reflection of their own emotional self-interest, your audience is rooting for you.*

**Visual Pause**   There may be times during your delivery that you want the audience's attention to switch from your verbal and visual delivery, to your verbal delivery alone. Perhaps you want to ask your learners a question, and have them consider their answers without access to any information on your slides. Perhaps you are about to make an important point, and want to fully engage their attention while you do so. In any case, do not hesitate to build in slide "pauses" to your presentation. In PowerPoint, this is easily accomplished by pressing the letter "B" on the keyboard, which will turn your screen to black [4, 5]. In other presentation software programs, you can build in a blank slide. This visual pause serves to focus learners' attention back on you and the words you say, and can provide a much needed visual break from slide progression. (See Chap. 8 for information about pauses when presenting virtually.)

Project your voice. Move your body. Refer to, but do not read, your slides. You are going to do great!

## 7.3   Post-Delivery (After)

At this point, you have invested an enormous amount of time and energy into all aspects of your presentation – crafting your visual delivery, practicing your verbal delivery, and developing your supplemental materials. Though it might be tempting to move on to something else, do not completely abandon your presentation just yet!

Ask yourself what worked well and what did not. Identify information that was unclear or unorganized. Make note of phrases or explanations that were particularly effective or particularly cumbersome. If you skipped or rushed through any slides, eliminate them. If you found yourself apologizing for a blurry image or complex figure, redo or revise it. If you ended up discussing content not included in your slides, consider adding an additional slide or slides.

Make revisions to your slides *now*, or use the slide notes function to indicate the changes that need to be made before you give the presentation again. The more work you do while the recent delivery is fresh in your mind, the better off you will be later when you want to deliver the same presentation again. Remember that high-quality slides are a reflection of your concern for the cognitive development of your learners. Send the message to students that the information you provide is important, and worth the time it takes to create, proof, and revise your presentation.

In order to not lose all of your hard work, be sure to archive it in such a way that it can be easily revisited [6]. Save your slide deck using descriptive information about when and where you presented it. Save any recording of your presentation in the same way. Together, your slides, recordings, and materials can serve as the basis of a teaching portfolio. A *healthy presentation* is one that also serves as a detailed record of your teaching practice, and goes a long way to keeping your CV updated and accurate in the long term.

**Summary Points**

- Before you begin your presentation, be sure to gather information about your audience and the presentation context.
- The best way to ensure a successful presentation is to practice it *out loud* ahead of time.
- Use the fact that your audience wants you to succeed as a way to decrease any public speaking anxiety.
- Be sure to save all slides, recordings, and materials in an organized way after your presentation.

# References

1. Alley M. The craft of scientific presentations: critical steps to succeed and critical errors to avoid. 2nd ed. New York: Springer; 2013.
2. Schraeder TL. Physician communication: connecting with patients, peers, and the public. Oxford: Oxford University Press; 2019.
3. Lang JM. Small teaching: everyday lessons from the science of learning. San Francisco: Wiley; 2016.
4. Atkinson C. Beyond bullet points: using Microsoft PowerPoint to create presentations that inform, motivate, and inspire (Bpg-other). Microsoft Press; 2005.
5. Duarte N. Slide: ology: the art and science of creating great presentations, vol. 1. Sebastapol: O'Reilly Media; 2008.
6. Nathans-Kelly T, Nicometo CG. Slide rules: design, build, and archive presentations in the engineering and technical fields, vol. 3. Hoboken: Wiley; 2014.

# Chapter 8
# Presenting Virtually

**Abstract**
This chapter provides tips to improve presentations that are delivered in a variety of virtual scenarios including in-person, recorded lectures; remote presenting to an in-person group; and fully remote. The various benefits and drawbacks of virtual presentations are discussed. *Healthy presentations* are defined as ones that facilitate learning for both in-person and remote learners, and that help you learn and grow as an educator.

In Chap. 1, I confessed that I love a good lecture. My second confession is that while I love a good lecture, I have never once made it through an hour-long webinar as a participant without simultaneously checking my email, texting, or otherwise multi-tasking. And I know I am not the only one.

These days we are all doing more teaching and presenting on virtual platforms. The beauty of online teaching is access – learners can access your content from their offices, bedrooms, and trains; via their phones, iPads, and laptops. When sessions are recorded, learners can access them asynchronously, sometimes weeks or months after the initial presentation. In Chap. 1, our hypothetical medical student "Ginny" used recorded medical school lectures to review content multiple times prior to exams. Playback of recordings can often be sped up or slowed down according to individual learner preference and comfort with the material. This can be especially helpful for learners with learning differences or disabilities.

Through virtual platforms, we have the potential to reach large numbers of learners. The registration numbers of the virtual sessions I run for faculty tend to be significantly greater than that of our in-person sessions. This makes sense – busy clinicians are hard pressed to find a free hour or hours in their day to engage in professional development. Clinical responsibilities start early, and evening professional development sessions conflict with family responsibilities. Sometimes, just the short drive from our hospitals to the medical school, and the brief search for parking are big enough barriers to prevent attendance, no matter how interested an individual may be in the content. Accessing material online, and potentially asynchronously, is very appealing.

> **Key Point**
> The advantage of virtual teaching is accessibility. The potential disadvantages include increased distraction and disengagement.

However, with remote access comes increased distraction, and a feeling of disconnection between presenter and audience. Audience members may also feel disconnected from one another. There may be a decrease in learner commitment to the activity at hand. The corollary to those increased registration numbers I mentioned above is an increase in attrition – far fewer individuals ultimately attend than register. "Accessibility" is accompanied by a certain *porousness* of attendance and attention – *the virtual modality that makes it easy for learners to appear also makes it easier for them to disappear, or to never show up at all.*

There is also an inherent tension between virtual platforms and the need to incorporate opportunities for active learning (see Chap. 4 for more on active learning). As virtual teachers, we need to work even harder to engage learners, and to create a sense of connection and community as we present. Below are several suggestions for how to do just that.

## 8.1   General Tips

**Ensure Facility with the Virtual Platform**  In order to focus on the more nuanced skills of engaging learners and creating connection, we need to be very facile with whatever platform we are using to present. It is not the goal of this chapter to provide technical guidance on every potential platform. There are innumerable online resources and YouTube videos available that can do that better and more comprehensively than I can here. My best advice is to practice ahead of time with any new platform or platform functionality in order to ensure as smooth a session as possible. If you encounter technical difficulties, try to keep calm. Remember that an anxious presenter leads to anxious and distracted learners. As much as possible, create a contingency plan ahead of time that accounts for various technical failures.

**Whenever Possible, Utilize a Co-Host**  Co-hosts can be invaluable for virtual sessions. Though not always available, co-hosts can help monitor the chat function and bring any questions to your attention. They can troubleshoot technical or logistical issues, and assign participants to breakout groups. Facilitating a virtual session, especially an interactive one with various technical components, is complex. If you are asked to present virtually, it is reasonable to inquire as to the availability of a co-host to help manage the session.

**Consider Shortening Individual Presentations** Overall presentation length may need to be shortened to account for the lack of physical presence, and for the visual fatigue inherent in virtual participation. Your 60-minute lecture may need to become three 20-minute lectures. Your 50-minute presentation may need to become 40 minutes long, with the addition of a handout as supplementary material.

> **Key Point**
> Virtual presentations may need to be shorter and faster paced than in-person presentations in order to facilitate attention and engagement.

**Increase Visual Pacing and Variety** Because remote learners are so easily distracted by other stimuli, individual presentations may need to involve a greater frequency of visual changes to engage their attention. The three, four, or five minutes you used to spend explaining one slide, may now be too long. Consider breaking up that information into smaller visual chunks that change at an increased pace during a virtual presentation. I am not advocating for a distillation of complex concepts into meaningless sound-bites, nor am I conflating attention with true engagement. I am advocating that your verbal discussion of complex concepts be accompanied by a succession of relevant, but more frequently changing, visuals.

The need for visual variety is perhaps most important for "webinars" that are slide and voice-over only, and that do not include any presenter presence. Evidence is mixed at this point as to the importance of a visible presenter on learning [1, 2]. However, it is undeniable that when slides are the only visual stimulus available to learners, we have to work harder to keep their attention.

The simplest way to achieve visual variety is to have text-based bullets appear one at a time rather than all at once, though there are a number of problems with over-reliance on bulleted lists (see Chap. 5) [3–5]. You can also call learner attention to various parts of a diagram through a series of arrows, circles, or highlights that appear on screen. One under-utilized strategy is to actually stop sharing your slides at various points during the presentation, engage with the audience directly with all of their attention focused on your face and voice, and then return to your slides.

**Number of Slides** An increased pace of slide changes will likely result in an increased number of slides per presentation. However, limits on slide numbers tend to be somewhat arbitrary, and are based on estimates of pacing that are often too slow, especially for virtual modalities. Arbitrary limits on the number of slides in a presentation can also have the unintended consequence of presenters shoving large amounts of information into a small proscribed number of slides! [6]. As long as your pacing is appropriate for the given modality, and you have practiced your presentation to make sure that your delivery stays within the given time-frame, the specific number of slides you use is irrelevant.

**Key Point**
The specific number of slides in your presentation is less important than the pace of your delivery. Practice your presentation out loud to ensure that your pace is appropriate for the content, and for the given time-frame of the talk.

## 8.2   Considerations for In-Person, Recorded Lectures

Even prior to COVID-19, much of undergraduate medical education had been moving to recorded lectures (Fig. 8.1) [7–9]. Pre-2020, these lectures were generally presented in person by faculty who ended up speaking to small numbers of medical students in largely empty lecture halls. Some faculty who are known to be excellent teachers might draw a crowd, but as the academic pressure builds across the first two years, and as USMLE Step 1 looms large, in-person attendance dwindles.

**Key Point**
We have a responsibility to help facilitate learning for all members of our audience – those in the room with us, and those accessing our presentations remotely.

Increasingly, students have tended to access recorded lectures on-line, and at times and in places (and potentially in pajamas), that worked for them. Faculty have expressed a great deal of dissatisfaction with this scenario, and rightly so. It can be incredibly disheartening to lecture to a mostly empty amphitheater. And it can be difficult to keep in mind all of the learners who are not in the room, but who will be accessing the presentation remotely. Yet we are responsible for those learners too, and we need to implement strategies that facilitate their learning as well.

**Use of Laser Pointers**  I have mixed feelings about laser pointers and their use during presentations in general. As the name suggests, they are designed to point to aspects of a projection that are out of reach. And yet as tools to direct audience attention they tend to be too anemic, too fleeting, and all too revealing of the occasional nervous, shaky hand. Generally we would be better off directing audience attention through the use of arrows, circles, or highlights that are incorporated directly into a slide.

The use of laser pointers is potentially even more problematic in lectures that are recorded. The light and movement of laser pointers are often not captured at all by the recording, thus making it difficult for remote learners to follow along. Some projection and recording systems require the use of specially connected slide advancers (which often come with laser pointer capacity), and thus the one you brought with you from your office to the lecture hall may not work. Before using a laser pointer, be sure to inquire as to whether or not it will actually feature in the recorded version of your talk.

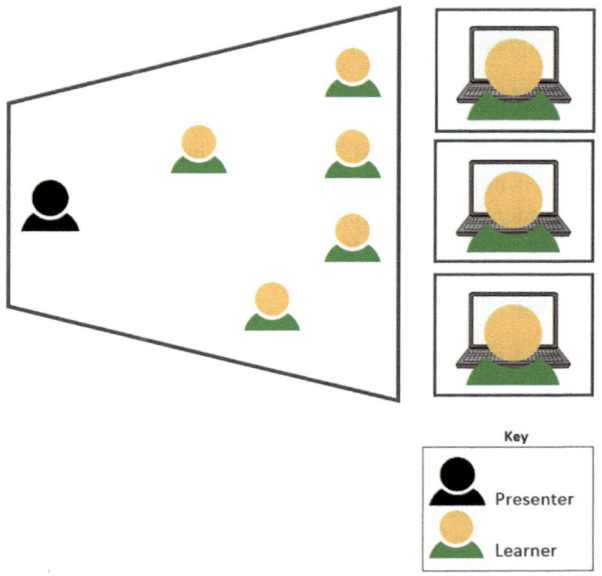

**Fig. 8.1** In-person, recorded lecture

*In-person, recorded lectures traditionally involved a presenter and a few learners in a large lecture hall. Other learners access the recording remotely, either via live stream, or as a recording*

**Staying in "Frame"** The cameras used to record in-person lectures are often located at the rear of large lecture halls. Thus the presenter may appear as a small figure in the distance, standing behind a lectern or moving back and forth in front of large projection screens. Other times the slide being projected forms one view, and a view of the presenter, perhaps just from the shoulders up, forms a second.

It is important that you inquire as to the visual arrangement of slides and presenter on the recorded version of your talk. I once viewed the recording of a talk I gave, only to realize after the fact that the view of my head was located in the top right-hand corner of each of my slides. Had I been aware of that spatial arrangement ahead of time, I would have ensured that none of the visuals on my slides were placed in that area.

For in-person lectures, you also run the risk of wandering out of the frame of the cameras, which can be disconcerting to your remote learners. Ideally, there will be specific areas taped off on the floor of the lecture hall that indicate your "in-frame" area. Even better, the cameras recording your talk will be visible, and close enough so that you can make occasional "eye contact" with your remote learners.

**The Sole Microphone** Most lecture halls are not equipped with sound systems that capture audience questions, and unless you are the featured speaker at a large event, it is unlikely that there are individuals running up and down the aisles with portable microphones. The only working mic in the room is probably attached to your shirt, or to the lectern. Therefore, yours will be the only voice that is automatically recorded. In order for remote learners to benefit from audience questions, *be sure to* *repeat each question before you answer it.* Otherwise remote learners will hear your answer, but not the question that prompted it.

Also, be aware that your conversations before and after your talk may be recorded as well. Perhaps you engaged in small talk with a colleague beforehand, or spent time chatting with learners afterward. Perhaps you lamented that the new generation of medical students is not as dedicated to their studies as they were in your day! The small number of students in the lecture hall may not have heard your comment, but your remote learners certainly did. It is always a good idea to check to make sure you turn off, remove, or move away from any microphones for any conversation you do not want recorded!

**Facilitating Active Learning**  Learners who are livestreaming your presentation will still be able to participate in electronic polling. They can also participate on their own in the "commitment" exercises that ask them to generate answers to the questions you pose (see Chap. 4). Remote learners can also complete and electronically submit any written assignments.

**Out-of-Class Information Transfer**  Because remote learners are not participating in in-person Q & A, you may need to consider additional ways to communicate with them. It may be tempting to respond to low student attendance with, "Well, they should have come to class." However, as mentioned above, there are real benefits of recorded lectures for learners who choose to access them asynchronously. Adult learning is particularly powerful when it is self-directed [10, 11], which may involve choosing when, how, and at what pace, to access material.

Our responsibility as educators extends beyond the classroom, and learners should not be penalized for opting for a virtual modality. For remote learners, we may need to dedicate more time to email communication, virtual office hours, or to creating more robust supporting materials that they can access asynchronously. (See Chap. 5 for additional information about the role of supplemental presentation material).

## 8.3  Considerations for Remote Presenting to an In-Person Group

There may be times when you are teaching from a remote location, but your learners are all physically in the same space (Fig. 8.2). For example, you may be giving a presentation from your office computer to a conference room in the hospital where a group of your fellows are gathered together. They can see you and/or your slides on the conference room projection screen, and you can see some or all of the group, though possibly from a distance.

When you are not physically present with your learners, it may be more difficult to develop connections with them. When an instructor is not in the same physical space, it is also incredibly difficult for learners to remain focused and resist distraction. For these reasons, it may be helpful to add additional structure to what may have previously been a more informal in-person interaction.

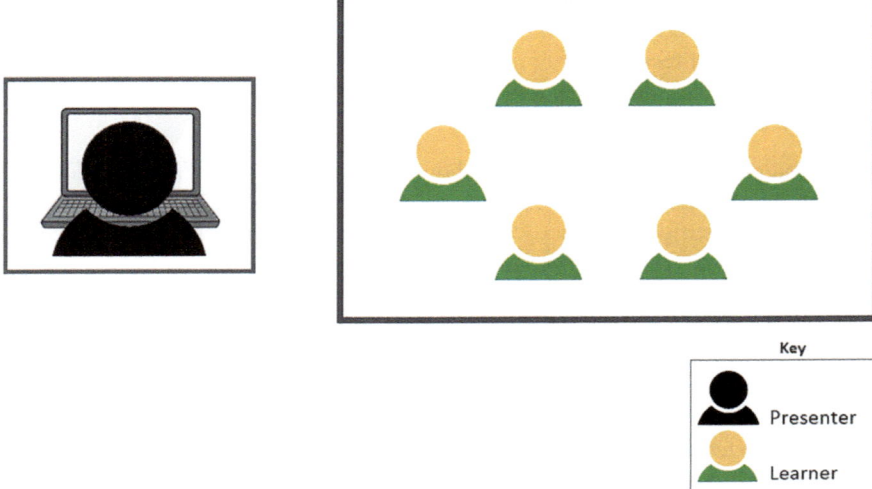

**Fig. 8.2** Remote presenting to an in-person group.

*Remote presenting to an in-person group involves presenting from an individual device, to a group of learners who are together in a shared physical space*

For example, you may have a presentation that you give to residents during each rotation. Usually you are together with a group of about eight residents in a small conference room. You have set up your didactic presentation such that you periodically turn to the group and ask questions. Traditionally one or two volunteers will provide the information, while the rest of the group listens. You have been able to move around the small space and make eye contact with each member of the group.

Now, however, your didactic session has been moved to a virtual platform. Your residents are located in two separate conference rooms on opposite sides of the hospital campus. You are presenting from your office and can see the two groups of masked residents from a distance on your monitor. It is unclear if the two groups can see each other. Unfortunately, sharing your screen makes it very difficult to see anyone at all as you present, as your slides take up the majority of your screen.

Your usual techniques of general questions, volunteered answers, and engagement through movement and eye contact, are not going to be sufficient in this scenario. Without individual devices, participants may not be able to take advantage of some of the virtual platform technology, such as chat or annotation functions. You will need other ways to connect with learners, encourage participation, and gauge understanding. I would encourage you to consider a more structured facilitation style, perhaps more structured than initially feels comfortable, in order to meet your goals.

> **Key Point**
> An increased level of structure is key to a well-facilitated virtual session.

**Structured Participation**  Utilize a facesheet if one is available, or ask participants to introduce themselves, and write down their names on a "seating chart." This way, even if you cannot recognize them visually, you have a record of their names. If you will be meeting with this group more than once, ask that participants sit in the same seats each time.

Call on participants by name throughout your presentation. While this does put learners "on the spot" it also establishes an expectation for attention and participation that is implicitly understood when you are physically present, but may need to be more explicitly established when presenting virtually.

Additionally, utilize the existing groups of participants. Pose a question and indicate that the groups should take a moment to discuss among themselves, and be ready to provide an answer. You can alternate between groups ("This question is for the group in Conference Room A, and the next one will be for the Conference Room C group."), or pose a question for both groups to consider, and then have everyone come back together to discuss.

Virtual Q & A requires an increased comfort with silence. Audio delays, fumbles with mute functions, and participation-reluctance mean that as a presenter, you need to provide additional time for learners to answer your questions. Structured participation can help mitigate some of these awkward delays and silences, and participants talking over one another, but be sure to wait an appropriate amount of time before rewording your question or otherwise moving on.

**Gauging Understanding**  It is exponentially more difficult to gauge learner understanding when you cannot see facial expressions or nodding of heads. You may miss confused looks or even raised hands when presenting remotely. Consider incorporating a mini-quiz into your presentation. You can ask participants to write down their answers informally, use a polling feature, or have learners actually log into a quiz platform to briefly answer a series of questions. Again, this may be more formal than you are comfortable with at least initially, but this level of structured assessment may be necessary to gauge learner understanding in a real way. Share your email at the end of your presentation and ask learners to contact you if they need clarification on concepts in your presentation.

**Maximizing your Presence**  Your physical presence has been reduced to a talking head on a screen. Your voice and body, once natural tools for engagement and relationship building, can now feel remote and potentially irrelevant. But as the presenter, you should never be irrelevant. The tools at your disposal are now your infectious enthusiasm for the topic, animated tone of voice, energetic hand gestures, and visually stimulating slide design (see Chap. 5). These tools are different than those you use when physically present with your learners, but they should be enhanced and maximized as much as possible during virtual presentations.

## 8.4   Considerations for Fully Remote Presenting

Fully remote presentation scenarios generally involve all individuals accessing the session on their own personal devices (Fig. 8.3). The benefits of this, compared with remote presenting to an in-person group, are not inconsequential. Fully remote teaching can ironically feel a bit less impersonal, especially if participants keep their video feeds on and are not wearing masks. Individual access means that each person is identifiable via a video image and/or the name that appears on their account.

In a fully remote mode of virtual presenting, you will still need to implement new ways to connect with learners, encourage participation, and gauge understanding. An increased focus on structured interaction is still my primary recommendation for fully remote sessions.

**Create Connection**   In order to bridge the sense of disconnection inherent in virtual teaching, introductions are even more important than they are during in-person teaching. Using learner names whenever possible can help to create a sense of community. The names that appear on individual accounts can be incredibly helpful in this regard. Because these names are so easily changed, presenters should feel free to ask participants to rename themselves if necessary.

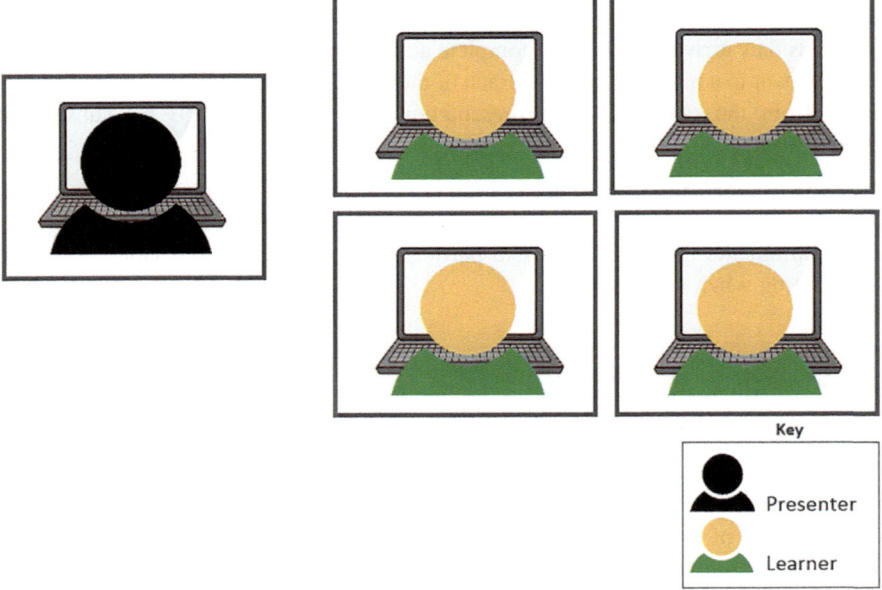

**Fig. 8.3**   Fully remote presenting.

*Fully remote presenting involves presenter and learners all on individual devices*

For example, a presenter might ask participants to take a moment to rename their account to "Preferred First Name.Year of Training" or "Full Name.Specialty" depending on the context of the presentation and what would facilitate connection and interaction. Consider asking individuals to rename themselves with phonetic pronunciations ("Emily: Eh-Meh-Lee") to assist in your ability to call on participants by name, or with preferred pronouns ("Emily.she/her/hers") to create a welcoming learning environment. I have participated in workshops where we were asked to rename ourselves to "First Name. How I am feeling today" which was a good conversation starter, but may not be appropriate for all academic settings.

**Session Logistics** Decide ahead of time how participants are going to enter your session. Are you going to use a "waiting room" function in order to check participant registration and prevent the type of "Zoom bombing" that occurred in 2020 as virtual teaching became more prevalent [12, 13]? If you decide against a waiting room, what measures will you take to avoid the awkward silence that occurs as participants join a session over the course of five or ten minutes? Be deliberate about your choices because in my experience, awkward silence at the outset of a presentation encourages participants to turn off their video feeds, and to begin engaging in other unrelated tasks as they wait. Recapturing already wandering attention makes the task of virtual teaching even more difficult.

If you are not going to utilize a "waiting room," consider integrating a "countdown" video (easily accessed on YouTube) into your slides so that participants know exactly when the presentation will begin. You can also engage participants in conversation as they arrive, ask them to complete a quick pre-session quiz, or to write down their answer to a relevant question. Each of these strategies encourages active engagement from the outset of your presentation, and sets the stage for subsequent participation.

**Explicit Expectations** In order to prepare your learners for an active virtual session, be sure to set explicit expectations. Consider ahead of time how you are going to communicate logistical details to participants, such as keeping video feeds on, and muting when not speaking.

> **Key Point**
> Ask learners to keep their video feeds on during discussions or small group work. Video feeds can be off when you are sharing your slides.

The issue of "video versus no video" is an interesting one. On the one hand, being able to see your learners helps you to feel connected, and helps participants to feel connected to one another, especially if the session includes a group discussion component. On the other hand, it can be exhausting to be "on camera" for long periods of time, and when you are sharing your slides, you cannot always see individual faces anyway. My recommendation is to make explicit the expectation that participants be able to turn off their video feeds during slide sharing, but turn their videos back on during any discussions or breakout sessions. You may also consider having participants choose a "virtual background" or blurred background while video feeds are on to reduce potential stigma or learner discomfort regarding living situations or personal environments.

**Participant Questions**   Decide ahead of time how you would like learners to ask questions. Explicitly encourage them to interrupt you verbally, or explicitly ask them to hold their questions until the end of your presentation. Indicate your preference that participants use the chat function, or raise their virtual hands. Feel free to label your session an "interactive workshop" or "discussion-based Grand Rounds" so that learners know going into the session that they will be expected to participate.

**Presenter Questions**   During virtual sessions, your use of questions to engage learners and to gauge their understanding may need to be more structured than you are used to, or comfortable with, during traditional in-person sessions. It may seem artificial or uncomfortable to call on participants instead of waiting for a volunteer to speak, but the reality is that remote participants are more easily able to fade into the background and wait for someone else to shoulder the burden of active participation than they can when you are physically present with them in a room. Virtual eye contact is more easily avoided than in-person eye contact, and video feeds can be turned off completely.

Discomfort with video sessions is real, and as I mentioned at the outset, I am not always the most active participant myself in virtual workshops. However, our goal is to facilitate learning, and participation can be key to that learning, even if it is occasionally reluctant in nature. At times, I have found that the most highly rated sessions are the ones that utilize learner time well and wisely through structured activities, "forcing" learners out of their comfortable, passive, modality. Inform participants ahead of time that you are going to be calling on individuals or groups so they can prepare appropriately.

In addition to asking questions, you will need to determine how you want your learners to provide answers to your questions. Certainly one option is to have them answer verbally. However, you can also utilize the polling function built-in to many virtual platforms. (See Chap. 4 for more information about audience response systems.) You can send learners to a shared document on which learners can write, though sharing a document can be difficult unless you have participant email addresses ahead of time. Alternately you can integrate a QR code into your slide which sends your participants to a URL where they will find a quiz, google form, website, etc., to facilitate sharing of information (Example 8.1).

**Example 8.1**  QR code (https://www.qr-code-generator.com/)

*Including a QR code on your slide as in Example 8.1 allows in-person and remote learners to access an online poll or other website using their smartphone's camera function. Free QR codes can easily be generated online.*

Many virtual platforms include an annotation function that allows participants to interact directly with the shared screen. They mark on a "whiteboard" or directly onto a slide as part of your presentation. The annotations can be "stamps," other marks, or text, all of which allow participants to provide answers to your questions in real time. You can use this annotation in creative ways.

**Participants can annotate to:**
- Indicate preference ("Which of these findings is more important clinically?")
- Select an option from a given list ("Mark which answer you think is correct.")
- Identify structures ("Put yellow stars on the occipital nerves.")
- Ask questions ("Use this space to write any remaining questions about areas that need clarification.")
- Draw processes ("Who can draw me a simple Krebs cycle?")
- Report back from breakout discussions ("What is on your differential?")

**Breakout Rooms**  Facilitating large group discussions in a virtual setting can be very difficult. Participants talk over one another, there are delays as individuals figure out how to unmute themselves. Suddenly the free exchange of ideas seems ponderous and exhausting for both participant and facilitator. Dividing your audience into smaller groups utilizing a breakout function is a good way to encourage interaction.

Again, these groups may need to be structured in ways that in-person groups do not. Be very clear with your learners about their tasks during the group discussion. Provide them with discussion questions ahead of time, and let them know what and how they will be asked to report out to the bigger group. Their first task may be to identify someone who will act as a reporter. Indicate exactly how long breakout groups will last, and what if any reminders you will be giving to the groups about time remaining.

The *bad news* is that well-crafted virtual presentations take more work to set up. Creating structure, setting explicit expectations, and using virtual technology to engage remote learners takes time and energy. In addition to the workload, our relative unfamiliarity with these platforms, and the fear of technological failures, can make the prospect of presenting virtually feel daunting.

I would argue however, that the attention we are now paying to our remote learners, and our concerns about whether they are in fact learning what we are teaching them, is attention that we should be paying to our traditional learners as well. We may have become complacent in the teaching strategies we use. Our traditional presentations could probably benefit from more structured participation. Our traditional learners could probably benefit from new efforts to gauge their understanding. The increasing prevalence of virtual sessions shines a light on improvements we can make to all of our teaching and presenting, regardless of modality.

The *good news* is that virtual presentations are almost always recorded, and recordings provide an opportunity for you to engage in some critical reflection about your strengths and weaknesses as a presenter. A *healthy presentation* is one that also helps you learn and improve as an educator! Do not hesitate to ask for a link to a recording so you can watch yourself present. In the comfort of your home or office, perhaps armed with a glass of wine (!), practice the "instructional empathy" I mention in Chap. 3 and become the audience for your own talk. Note what went well, and any areas you may want to improve. We are all life-long learners, and with enough honest critique, presenting skills, even virtual ones, are very amenable to improvement.

**Summary Points**
- Although virtual education allows for increased access, it can also lead to increased distraction and disengagement on the part of the learners.
- Virtual presentations may require a shorter duration and more frequently changing visuals.
- As biomedical educators we have a responsibility to facilitate learning for in-person and remote learners.
- Considerations for in-person, recorded lectures include potential avoidance of laser pointer use, an awareness of what is being recorded, and an understanding of how recordings appear to remote learners.
- Considerations for remote presenting to an in-person group include the need for additional session structure and explicit expectations around participation.

- Considerations for fully remote presenting include the need for additional session structure, explicit expectations around participation, and intentional focus on the creation of connection and community.
- While virtual presentations require a great deal of work to set up, they also represent an opportunity for us to improve our teaching practice.

## References

1. Wang J, Antonenko PD. Instructor presence in instructional video: effects on visual attention, recall, and perceived learning. Comput Hum Behav. 2017;71:79–89.
2. Wang J, Antonenko P, Dawson K. Does visual attention to the instructor in online video affect learning and learner perceptions? An eye-tracking analysis. Comput Educ. 2020;146:103779.
3. Duarte N. Slide: ology: the art and science of creating great presentations, vol. 1. Sebastapol: O'Reilly Media; 2008.
4. Mayer RE. Multimedia learning. Cambridge, Cambridge University Press; 2009.
5. Tufte ER. The cognitive style of PowerPoint. New York: AP/Wide World Photos; 2003.
6. Atkinson C. Beyond bullet points: using Microsoft PowerPoint to create presentations that inform, motivate, and inspire (Bpg-other). Microsoft Press; 2005.
7. Emanuel EJ. The inevitable reimagining of medical education. JAMA. 2020;323(12):1127–8.
8. Ikonne U, Campbell AM, Whelihan KE, Bay RC, Lewis JH. Exodus from the classroom: student perceptions, lecture capture technology, and the inception of on-demand preclinical medical education. J Am Osteopath Assoc. 2018;118(12):813–23.
9. Prober CG, Heath C. Lecture halls without lectures—a proposal for medical education. N Engl J Med. 2012;366(18):1657–9.
10. Knowles MS. Self-directed learning: a guide for learners and teachers. Chicago: Association Press; 1975.
11. Merriam SB, Caffarella R, Baumgartner S. Learning in adulthood: A comprehensive guide. 3rd ed. San Francisco: Jossey-Bass; 2007.
12. Hern A. Trolls exploit zoom privacy settings as app gains popularity, GUARDIAN (Mar. 27, 2020 8:23 AM), https://www.theguardian.com/technology/2020/mar/27/trolls-zoom-privacy-settingscovid-19-lockdown, FORBES (Mar. 27, 2020 11:19 AM).
13. Mohanty M, Yaqub W. Towards seamless authentication for zoom-based online teaching and meeting. arXiv preprint arXiv:200510553. 2020;

# Chapter 9
# Implementing Change

**Abstract**
This chapter outlines the steps we need to take to implement improvements to our presentations. It includes additional tips about how to get started, and about concrete areas of focus such as the identification and preservation of key images, and organization of our materials. Finally, it summarizes the characteristics of *healthy presentations*.

We have established by now (I hope) that we must improve our presentations in order to properly do our job as biomedical educators. But change is hard, and in Chap. 2, I acknowledged that it can feel risky to deviate from our educational and professional norms. It can also seem like an insurmountable task to think about overhauling every presentation you have already developed, or starting from scratch in new and different ways with presentations you have yet to craft. For novice presenters, these challenges can feel even more overwhelming.

While I firmly believe that improved presentations will lead to improved learning, I do not expect busy clinicians and scientists to suddenly become graphic designers, or inspirational TED Talk speakers, upon finishing this book. Your dense and detailed content will still need to be presented. Photographs of sunsets and rock sculptures will still probably not find a home in your slide deck. You may still rely on text-heavy slides to get certain concepts across. That is okay. Do not sacrifice "better" in pursuit of "great." Start small, with one new or existing talk. Choose a talk that is low-stakes, not one that is part of a job interview, or in front of a national audience.

To revise an existing talk, follow these five basic steps (Fig. 9.1):

1. *Select content to support learning objectives:* Determine if you are happy with the overall selection of content. Check to make sure that the information you

include supports the major concepts you want your audience to learn. Think critically about the *amount* of information you include, and whether or not a portion of it could be relocated to a handout or some other kind of supplemental material (Chaps. 3 and 5).

2. *Lead and engage:* Consider the need to lead and engage your audience. Check to make sure that you are "holding their hands" by referring to an outline or other organizer as you transition between topics. Where appropriate, add a brief activity, even a simple question and answer session (remember to also <u>W</u>ait and <u>D</u>eflect!), to facilitate active learning and keep your audience engaged. Remember that virtual presentations require even more effort to keep learners engaged (Chaps. 2, 3, 4, and 8).

3. *Review for inclusivity:* Review your content for inclusive images and language. Confirm that you can explain how and why race and other variables related to patient identity feature in the data you present (Chap. 6).

4. *Improve slide design:* Identify opportunities to improve your slide design. You do not have to redesign the entire presentation. If your current theme is very busy, you can change it to a plain white background with one click. Otherwise, spend a few minutes searching for simple changes to make on individual slides – delete clip-art, enlarge diagrams, and enhance bulleted lists with the use of shapes, color, and other visual and conceptual illustrations (Chap. 5).

5. *Practice:* And finally, practice, practice, practice. Each time you run through your talk, you will find new improvements to make, and gain new confidence in your ability to facilitate learning with your delivery (Chap. 7).

You may actually find it easier to design a new presentation using the steps above than to revise an existing one, as we tend to have a hard time really "seeing" presentations we have given multiple times.

When creating a new talk from scratch, the steps are much the same, though more time should be spent on the first step as you map out learning objectives and lecture parameters *prior* to opening any slide presentation software. When trying out slide design tips and presentation strategies on a new talk, be sure that the topic is one with which you are comfortable, so you are not learning content and figuring out how to teach it at the same time.

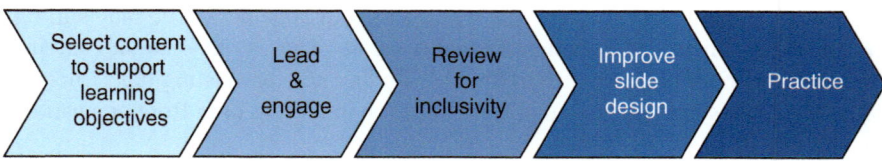

**Fig. 9.1** Steps for implementing change

**Identify Key Images**  Other things you can do to implement change include identifying "go to" images that you find yourself including in multiple presentations. If these images (including tables, graphs, photographs, etc.) are of poor quality or overly complex, it may be worth recreating or replacing them now for the future. Consider investing in a paid subscription to an image library if you have difficulty finding high-quality images to use.

**Gather Your Materials**  You might also consider creating a website using a learning management system such as Canvas, Blackboard, or Google Classroom in which you can post materials and articles you cite frequently. The site can act as a repository for your supplemental materials, and for pdf copies of your slides. Start pairing slide decks with these sets of supplemental materials in organized folders so that you can come back to them again and again over time.

**Label Clearly**  Be sure to save every slide deck you create using descriptive information about when and where you delivered the presentation. This information will be invaluable when making further revisions and improvements to the presentation down the line. It can also serve as the basis of a teaching portfolio, and make it easier to keep your CV updated with all of your teaching and presenting activities.

Presentation quality matters. High-quality presentations lead to efficient and effective learning, which in turn can lead to improved clinical practice and learner satisfaction. You may also find your instructional practice increasingly rewarding as you engage with your audience in new and different ways.

**Healthy presentations…**
- Have the *facilitation of learning* as their single and central goal.
- Help our learners to effectively and efficiently comprehend and retain the information we provide.
- Appropriately align content to the audience and advance specific learning objectives.
- Include opportunities for *active* learning.
- Are visually varied and engaging, and combat the shortcomings of presentation software default designs.
- Communicate an updated understanding of race as a social construct, and help learners construct new knowledge that is accurate and inclusive.
- Serve as a detailed record of your teaching practice.
- Help you learn and improve as an educator.

As clinicians, educators, and researchers, it is our responsibility to teach to the best of our abilities. Use just a bit of your very limited professional time to experiment with creating *healthy presentations.*

**Summary Points**
- It can feel daunting to revise existing presentations, or to begin crafting a new presentation in a different way.
- Start small, with a low-stakes talk and familiar content.
- Engage in five basic steps when revising existing presentations: (1) Select content to support your learning objectives. (2) Lead and engage. (3) Review for inclusivity. (4) Improve slide design. (5) Practice, practice, practice!
- Identify key images you will use over and over, gather your materials in one place, and label all of your teaching endeavors clearly.

# Index

**A**
Active cognition verbs, 28
Active learning
    case-based learning, 33, 34
    definition, 27, 28
    mini-assignments
        haiku, 33
        3-question quiz, 33
        quick-write, 32
        truths and a lie, 33
    questioning
        audience members' commitment, 30
        audience response systems, 29
        goal, 28
        transform "Q & A" to "Q D & A", 29
        transform "Q & A" to "Q W &
            A", 28, 29
        turn & talk activity, 30
    workshop elements
        fishbowl exercise, 31
        opinion spectrum, 32
        role play, 31
Annotation, 93, 98
Association for Medical Education in Europe's
        (AMEE), 29
Audience goodwill, 83
Audience response systems, 29

**B**
Backwards design, 14
Biomedical presentations, 8, 9
Blackboard, 103
Branching-plot clinical case, 34
Breakout rooms, 98

Bulleted lists
    template slide-comparison
        of clinical findings across slides, 52
        of diseases across slides, 51
    traditional bulleted list, 44–46, 48, 50
    use of, 43
    visual image, 50
    visual mnemonics, 55

**C**
Canvas, 103
Cliff Atkinson's Beyond Bullet Points, 17
Clinical language, 68
Clip-art images, 58, 67
Cognitive load, 39, 57, 60
Co-hosts, 88, 89
Color scheme, 57
Color, space, and variety of images, 60, 61
Commitment, audience response, 30
Common slide design, 39, 40
Content-rich slides, 8
Core concepts, 14, 15
Crafting a talk
    active verbs usage, 15
    appropriate teaching strategies, 15
    beginnings
        hook, 18, 19
        rest of the slides, 20
        self-introduction, 17
    defining core concepts, 14, 15
    inherited slides, 16
    middles
        endings, 25
        outline, 21–23

Crafting a talk (*cont.*)
    parameters, 21
    slide numbers, 24
    understanding learners, 13, 14
Cue cards, 10
CV, 84

**D**
Delivery
    in preparation (before)
        know the context, 82, 83
        know your learners, 81, 82
    in the moment (during)
        audience goodwill, 83
        visual pause, 83, 84
    post-delivery (after), 84
Didactic session, 93
Disclosure, 76, 77
Discussion-based Grand Rounds, 97
Disengagement, 99
Distraction, 88, 92, 99

**E**
Educational presentations, 17
Ethnicity, 63, 65, 68, 69
Exceptional lectures, 2

**F**
Facesheet, 94
"Faithful" visual representations, 59
Fishbowl exercise, 31
Fully remote presentation, 95

**G**
Good slide design, 9
Good teaching, 9, 10
Google Classroom, 103

**H**
Haiku, 33
Heterogeneous images, 64
High quality presentations, 103
High-quality slides, 84
Homogeneous images, 64
Hook, 18, 19

**I**
Improvements in presentations
    gathering materials together, 103
    identifying key images, 103
    labelling clearly, 103
    revising an existing talk
        improving slide design, 102
        leading and engaging audience, 102
        practicing, 102
        review for inclusivity, 102
        selecting content to support learning
            objectives, 101
Inclusive and antiracist teaching, 68
Inclusive language, 67
Inclusive teaching practices, 63
"In-frame" area, 91
Inherited slides, 16
In-person, recorded lecture, 91
Instructional empathy, 13, 25
Interactive workshop, 97

**L**
Laser pointers, 90
Learner engagement, 9, 10
Learner-centered, 10
Learning management system, 103
Learning objectives, 14
Learning paradigm, 10
Lectures, 10

**M**
Medical and health professions
    education, 10
Microphones, 91, 92
Mock code program, 2
Multimedia instruction, 39
Myths
    audience members knowledge, 9
    biomedical presentations, 8, 9
    good teaching, 9, 10
    professional presentations, 8
    traditional presentations, 7, 8

**O**
One-minute paper, 32
Online teaching, 87
Opinion spectrum, 32

**P**

Polling feature, 94
Poor quality visual image, 59
Poster design, 42
Professional presentations, 8
Public speaking, 7

**Q**

Q & A process, 28, 29
Q D & A process, 29
QR code, 98
Quality, 3, 5, 6
3-Question quiz, 33
Quick-write, 32
Q W & A process, 28

**R**

Race
    prevalence by racial category, 73–75
    as risk factor, 69–72
Recording lectures, 87
Reviewing slides for diversity and inclusion
    citations review, 68, 69
    clip-art, 67
    homogeneous and heterogeneous
        images, 64
    inclusive and antiracist teaching, 68
    language and terminology, 67, 68
    prevalence by racial category, 73–75
    race as a risk factor, 69–73
    range of possible edits, 75
        definition of terms, 77, 78
        disclosure, 76, 77
        explain (or eliminate), 75, 76
    single "representative" image, 66
    use of diverse images, 65
Revising an existing talk
    improving slide design, 102
    leading and engaging audience, 102
    practicing, 102
    review for inclusivity, 102
    selecting content to support learning
        objectives, 101
Revisions, to slides, 84
Role play, 31

**S**

Saving slides, 84
Self-introduction, 17
Slide design

anatomy of presentation, 37–39
assertion-evidence design, 41, 42
color, space, and variety of images, 60, 61
common slide design, 39, 40
simple is better, 55
    contrasting colors, 57
    fonts, 56
    quantitative "rules, 56
    templates, 56
text and visual elements, 59, 60
using text differently
    bulleted lists (*see* Bulleted lists)
    geographical concepts, 53
    timelines and process, 52, 53
    visual mnemonics, 54
visual elements, 58
Slide numbers, 24
Slides-as-cue-cards, 10
Social construct, 78
Software program, 17, 25
Structured participation, 94
Succinct lectures, 2
Supplemental materials, 38, 39

**T**

Teacher-delivered, 10
Teaching portfolio, 84
Teaching strategies, 14–16
Text and visual elements, 59, 60
Text-based slide decks, 7
Traditional academic lectures, 6
Traditional content outline, 22
Traditional instruction paradigm, 10
Traditional presentations, 7, 8
Truths and a lie, 33
Turn and talk activity, 30

**V**

Verbal delivery, 37, 39, 61
"Video *versus* no video", 96
Virtual background, 97
Virtual eye contact, 97
Virtual presentation
    advantages, 99
    co-hosts, 88, 89
    disadvantages, 99
    ensuring facility, 88
    fully remote presentation
        breakout rooms, 98, 99
        creating connection, 95, 96
        explicit expectations, 96, 97

Virtual presentation (*cont.*)
    participant questions, 97
    presenter questions, 97
    session logistics, 96
  in-person, recorded lectures
    active learning, 92
    "in-frame" area, 91
    laser pointers, 90
    microphones, 91, 92
    out-of-class information transfer, 92, 93
  number of slides, 89
  remote presenting to in-person group, 92
    didactic session, 93
    gauging understanding, 94
    maximizing presence, 94
    structured participation, 94
  shortening individual presentations, 89
  visual pacing and variety, 89

Virtual Q & A, 94
Virtual workshops, 97
Visual delivery, 37, 61
Visual elements, 58
Visual mnemonics, 54, 55
Visual pacing, 89
Visual pause, 83, 84
Visual persuasion, 17
Visual variety, 89

**W**
Webinars, 89
Well-designed slides, 8

**Z**
Zoom bombing, 96